BORDERS OF TIME
Life in a Nursing Home

Narrative text by Walter H. Crandall
Photographs by Rob Crandall

With the editorial assistance of Susan Page York

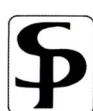

Springer Publishing Company
New York

Copyright © 1990 by Walter H. Crandall (text) and Rob Crandall (photographs)

Published by Springer Publishing Company, Inc.

All rights reserved

No part of this publication may be reproduced, stored in a retrieval system, or transmitted in any form or by any means, electronic, mechanical, photocopying, recording, or otherwise, without the prior permission of Springer Publishing Company, Inc.

Springer Publishing Company, Inc.
536 Broadway
New York, NY 10012

90 91 92 93 94/5 4 3 2 1

Library of Congress Cataloging-in-Publication Data

Crandall, Walter H.
    Borders of time : life in a nursing home / narrative text by Walter H. Crandall ; photographs by Rob Crandall ; with the editorial assistance of Susan Page York.
       p.   cm.
    Bibliography: p.
    Includes index.
    ISBN 0-8261-6890-6
    1. Nursing homes—Oregon. I. Crandall, Rob, 1956–   . II. York, Susan Page.
III. Title.
RA997.5.O7C73 1989
362.1'6'09795—dc19   89-6017
                                                                                                    CIP

Printed in the United States of America

For Kathy
───────────
and our parents

ACKNOWLEDGMENTS

We are grateful to Barbara Watkins, Vice President and Senior Editor, Springer Publishing Company, for having the courage to bring this project to fruition and for her invaluable criticism, and to Kathleen Kelly, Editorial/Production Manager at Springer, for her meticulous attention and care in guiding the project through the production stages.

Our special thanks to our editor, Susan Page York, for her friendship, commitment to the project, and highly imaginative criticism, which made an enormous contribution.

Our thanks to the residents, staff and families of the nursing home; to Stephen Levien for his friendship, his research assistance, and for his criticism; to Lonnie Perry for his friendship and unwavering devotion to nursing home residents; to Katherine Chavigny, Ph.D., Director of Medical Education and Science, American Medical Association, for her encouragement and support; to Robert Baker for his help; to Prescott Thompson, M.D., for his interest and encouragement; to Jane Kirschling, R.N., D.N.S., Assistant Professor, Aging Family Nursing, Oregon Health Sciences University, School of Nursing, for her encouragement and help; and to Rob Ail, Sales Manager, American Business Machines, for his generous help.

FOREWORD

While much is now being written about nursing homes, this book is different. It brings us inside the lives of the people who live and work in a long-term care institution. Through the efforts of cousins Walter and Rob Crandall, we see and hear the laundry supervisor and the social worker, the nurse, the nurse's aide and the physician, and most of all, the residents themselves. This book is a window on their dreams and daily frustrations. It manages, through an artful blend of words and photographs, to overcome our denial of the realities of age or illness or place. This book is about the rich and complex human world that exists in nursing homes. It helps us appreciate the deep rewards to be had in getting to know those who live in nursing homes. By understanding more fully the experiences of those who must spend their last days in institutions, we may be moved to work to improve the quality of life and the quality of nursing home care. This sensitive and moving book should be especially appreciated by those who work in the field of aging.

ROBERT N. BUTLER, M.D.
The Mount Sinai Medical Center
New York City

CONTENTS

      Introduction ———————— xiii

I.   **Prologue** ———————————— 1

II. **Links Forged and Broken** ——— 15

    Pat and Hazel
    Wilbur and Cecil
    Donnabelle and Genevieve
    Georgia
    Frank and Rosa
    Minnie

III. **Caretakers** ————————— 41

    Shirley
    Ken
    Richard
    Lonnie
    Carol
    Rose
    Alice
    Twenty-two Times

IV. **Outsiders** ————————— 55

    Television
    Santa Claus
    Senior Producer, Town Hall
    Father Howard
    Funeral Director
    Brother Loren

V. **Reflections** ———————— 65

    Flying East
    He Was a Good Man

    Horatio
    Nobody Left
    A Trailer House in the Country
    I Got Plenty to Eat
    Women Get Pushed Around
    Herding Cattle
    Hell of a Beautiful Woman
    Baby
    A Bouquet of Flowers
    She Knew
    Fifty Feet
    Vergie

VI. **The Chill** ————————— 81

    I've Been Feeling Just Fine
    Something Snapped
    An Old Bull's Neck
    They Do It to Old People
    I Don't Want to Die
    He Died Up in 18
    After Midnight
    Waiting

VII. **Keeping On, Moving On** ——— 101

    Death Hath No Terror
    Mom Really Believed
    Recovery
    I'll Just Whittle Away to Nothing
    Then Trumpets Sound
    Those Were Grandma's Qualities

About the Authors ———————— 115

Introduction

When I moved out to the West Coast, I became involved with the Gray Panthers' Nursing Home Task Force. As part of my work I wrote a consumer guide, *Living in Oregon's Nursing Homes,* with almost no experiential background. Two members of the Task Force—Shirley and Lonnie who worked together at the same nursing home—urged me on a number of occasions to visit their home. I always found an excuse not to visit. Oddly enough, I thought I was able to form expert opinions on the subject without feeling the need to spend much time in nursing homes.

In one of those fortunate twists of fate, a gust of wind blew the illustrations for the guide out the window of the graphic designer's office. The graphic designer refused to start over again. After exhausting a number of possibilities, I asked Shirley, the Director of Nursing, if my cousin Rob Crandall, a photographer, could photograph some of the residents. She agreed. One thing led to another: I gained permission to be admitted to the nursing home as a mock patient for a week; I worked as a nurse's aide for three months; and somewhere along the line Rob and I decided to pursue a book project. We spent more than two years photographing and talking to the residents.

When Rob and I first started visiting the nursing home, we didn't see the residents so much as feel them as tiny bits of muscular tension. The seeming invisibility of the residents distanced us from them, allowing us a slower transition into the life of the nursing home than they themselves had been granted. Still, we experienced daily some aspect of growing old that could not be ignored.

During one of our early visits, a man from South hall, the heavy care ward, broke the fragile truce between body odors and disinfectant when he evacuated his bowels during the middle of a concert given by a ladies auxiliary group. That unmistakable smell pierced the surroundings: our noses twitched, our eyes filled with shame. The stench confirmed our fear that the nursing home is a place for people who have lost control of their bodies. Worse, it confirmed that just as the body is helpless when life begins, so it is at the end.

In the beginning, we expended a considerable amount of energy trying to gather interviews and visual material for the book we wanted to produce about how terrible it is to be in a nursing home, and how nursing homes need improvement. We wanted to warn: Watch out folks! This could happen to you. But no matter how hard we tried to keep the nursing home at bay and carry out our purpose, we were always rebuked. There was no getting along with the place except on its own terms. And the stake was bigger than we had anticipated. We began to realize that if we failed to see an inherent value in the people we talked with, and saw the home only as an institution that sustains what is considered shameful and forbidden, then that said more about ourselves than it did about the nursing home. It could not be viewed as just a piece of pathology to be understood. Nor was it possible to just record its surface reality.

We began to hear their voices, at first so unsettling and mysterious— "Nurse, nurse, I love you. Give me a cookie . . . One for you and one for me." Messages with meaning, not addlepated ramblings of the old. As their lives took on form and content, some of our backed-up guilt and obscure hostility were released, freeing us to move across to the volatile world of human feelings.

As Rob and I moved about in the nursing home, we began to talk to the residents in a different way, asking a multitude of questions about their lives and experiences. Gradually some of the residents began to talk to us more openly. We heard some say, with evident astonishment, that their senses sometimes played tricks on them, that their world was askew. It is 1923—not decades later; they are footloose and fancy-free, not spirits entombed in decrepit bodies. When they look in the mirror, they find it hard to believe how time has altered them. Etched in the tissue-thin flesh of their faces are all of their losses. The husband, affectionately referred to as "a good man," died years ago, leaving his widow in a society that no longer knows what to do with her. Children, still visible in frayed snapshots, are now adults, scattered around the country. The bankbook, like the cupboard of an unlived in house, lies bare and forgotten.

With new appreciation we hear their stories. How they daydream—shut their eyes, take a deep breath, and float backward through time to a place where they believe they had lived simply, unburdened by problems and fears, or where they had been able to find a way to ease their difficulties. Many return to their childhoods. The memory of wandering in the woods, gathering Indian Pipes and violets, and making birch tree baskets in the shape of birds and butterflies.

Others talked about the future. As a young man, Arthur had gone to Alaska with the simple confidence that he would realize his dream of starting a construction business: some sixty-five years later, with death approaching, he agonized about the national debt, concerned that if left unchecked it could have a devastating effect on his grandchildren and great-grandchildren. In his day, you paid your debts, you took care of your family, and you didn't owe anybody—it was as simple as that. Arthur believed, as if it were written in stone, that each generation has the obligation to act responsibly for the succeeding generations.

Listening to their stories, we are reminded that most of the residents were born between 1895 and 1905, during a time when the country was undergoing a sweeping transformation. Rural America, though still very much a part of the national psyche, was beginning to lose its grip on the American imagination, giving way to the forces of urbanization and industrialization. For many this was an exciting time, bringing a sense of hope and promise that their individual lives would assume an ease never before imagined. But it seemed that what was so remarkable to the people we talked with was not all the technological triumphs they had witnessed, but how fast things had changed.

Looking out the big plate glass window in North dining room at the surge and blur of the traffic, some of the women would talk sadly about the days when the pace of life seemed set to the clanging of the trolley. Then their eyes would twinkle as they imagined themselves strolling down main street, exchanging pleasantries with the shopkeepers, all of whom they knew by name.

As we found out, the complexity of life doesn't necessarily shut down once you are at a nursing home. In some ways it is intensified. Often alone and with little or no prospects for the future, many of the residents reach out for a last chance at human contact. How this is played out gives a poignancy to the nursing home that is rarely perceived by outsiders.

Each person we talked with had their own way of dealing with their situation. For every crisis, every fear, Essie would reel off a piece of Biblical wisdom. On the subject of death, her voice would crack with emotion, lapse into a reverent stillness, then suddenly come crashing down like thunder: "Man that is born of a woman is of a few days!" Then she would raise her hand in testimony, assuring everybody that, "death hath no terror."

Like many of the residents without Essie's strong faith, we found ourselves struggling for some kind of resolution to those unsettling, but unavoidable questions about the character of love, our obligation to others, why people suffer, and the meaning of death. Those residents who had resolved these questions seemed less affected by the often chaotic, sometimes soul-numbing environment.

So much of the nursing home is defined by the paralyzing rhythm of one day unfolding grudgingly into another. After a while, yesterday, today, and tomorrow become almost indistinguishable from each other, creating a kind of time warp. In a place like this people can spend almost all of their waking hours in reflection. Here, time—if you allow it—can easily eat away at the rational world, stirring up old phantoms and creating new ones. Especially vulnerable are the women who suffer in silence—the ones who rarely complain and who swear you to secrecy when they do, nervously looking around, like a burrow creature just climbing out of its hole. They are the ones who will lie in bed at midnight, wringing wet with their sweat, wondering whether they are wanted or belong in this world, and fearful that perhaps there might not be a place for them in the next.

For those residents who have not outlived their relatives, the way they handle their predicament in part reflects the way their families respond to them. Ramona, a resident, described the place as "a mansion of broken hearts with God in the offing."

Those friends and relatives who visited on a regular basis are the ones who gave us some insight into what had happened. They had the capacity to work through their intense feelings about placing their loved ones in a nursing home, thus accepting their loved one's condition as well as the constraints of the nursing home. They were able to form alliances with the staff instead of working against them. But what really set them apart was something more elusive; it spoke to the attitude that love isn't enough. Even when it is inconvenient to visit your parent, spouse, or other relative, or no matter how ambivalent you may feel about them, you just do it. It's your duty.

* * *

The nursing home has the fragile and everchanging ecology of a tidal pool. For a while the home will be on a roll, fully staffed, and everything will be going smoothly. There is a relaxed, give-and-take relationship between the staff and residents. You can see it on a Saturday night in Room 56, where Lawrence Welk's champagne music entertains three dowagers. Barbara, a young nurse who showed up at the Halloween party in the home dressed as Wonder Woman, enters the room; a frail looking woman in a housedress smiles and stands up. They begin to waltz to the music. The woman is surprisingly agile as she whirls Barbara around the tiled floor. Near the end of the number, one of the woman's stockings falls down to her ankle. Embarrassed, she stops dancing and mutters to herself in German. With a little ingenuity, Barbara attaches rubber bands to her stocking. "Let's Polka," says Barbara, when the band changes tempo. The woman blushes. Her friends start giggling like school kids, urging her to dance, but the woman refuses. A polka is a bit too risque for her.

Things change. A number of key staff leave: the Director of Nursing; several aides who had earned the trust of the patients; a cook who could really cook. The place turns mean. A barometer are the ten to fifteen residents on South who usually catnap along the hall before dinner. When things turn sour, they wake up like hornets, agitated and buzzing at each other.

The aides are the ones who are responsible for putting out these brush fires. The work is both physically and emotionally demanding; the pay is just above minimum wage. Most aides are women. After a brief training period, the new aides—some of whom are young kids with spotty employment records—are thrown into the rough and tumble of nursing home life. Some are vulnerable themselves, as much dependent on the old people as the old are dependent on them. They treat some of the residents as if they were their children, scolding them when they are naughty, laughing at their idiosyncracies, comforting them when they are ill, mourning them when they die. They balk at the professionals who advise them not to become emotionally involved. What do the professionals know about love, they ask.

The professionals, with more experience, better understand how to maintain their emotional balance. Maryanne, the activity director, knows that during Christmas she will have trouble fitting in all of the groups who want to visit or entertain the residents and whom she can't refuse. But during the rest of the year she will, as she says, "Be banging down the doors trying to get community groups to visit us." Still, she stays on. Richard, the house physician, initially felt that he had to apologize to his colleagues for practicing medicine in a nursing home. He and Maryanne, and others like them, understand that society places very little value in the work they do; there has been no tradition and no honor in taking care of the elderly. Yet these people continue, with compassion and strength, to do their work well.

As I found out, strangers taking care of strangers can lead to precarious, sometimes explosive, and ambiguous relationships. I learned this, when I worked as a nurse's aide, from a blind and confused old man whose voice had a lyrically disturbing quality. His room was at the end of south hall.

The old man didn't like to be touched; every time I changed him there was a skirmish. It would start just as soon as I crossed the threshold of his room (there was nothing wrong with the man's hearing). His body would stiffen, as if rigor mortis had set in. As I approached his bed, he would grasp the top sheet with his bony hand and hold on for dear life, all the while cursing and pleading with me in Italian. The battle of Room 76 had commenced. The more I tried to pry the sheet loose, the more he thrashed about. One day I outfoxed him. Ever so quietly I tiptoed into the room and, in one clean jerk, snatched away the covers. He didn't take this lying down, as I found out on my next tour. In a declaration of war, he had smeared excrement all over his bed.

I found the old man troublesome. Whether he meant to be or not, he was a kind of gadfly. I came to see that there was something wrong in our relationship. I was treating him as an object of pity and he was telling me he didn't like it.

Some months later, Rob and I are standing by the cigarette machine at 3:00 A.M. in North dining room, idly staring out the big plate glass window at the empty street. The place is silent, as if time were lying still. Soon streaks of daylight will emerge from the swirl of darkness, heralding another day of people aging. I hear a loud voice which has the broken and rough melody of a sea chantey, resounding throughout North hall. Then silence returns. Early morning thoughts. I think about the old Italian man. For a moment I imagine that I am old and alone amidst strangers, sitting mournfully on the edge of my bed. Here the old man and I are on equal footing. Despite our differences we share a common identity in our need for food, shelter, warmth, respect, and love. We are truly brothers travelling together through the borders of time.

I. Prologue

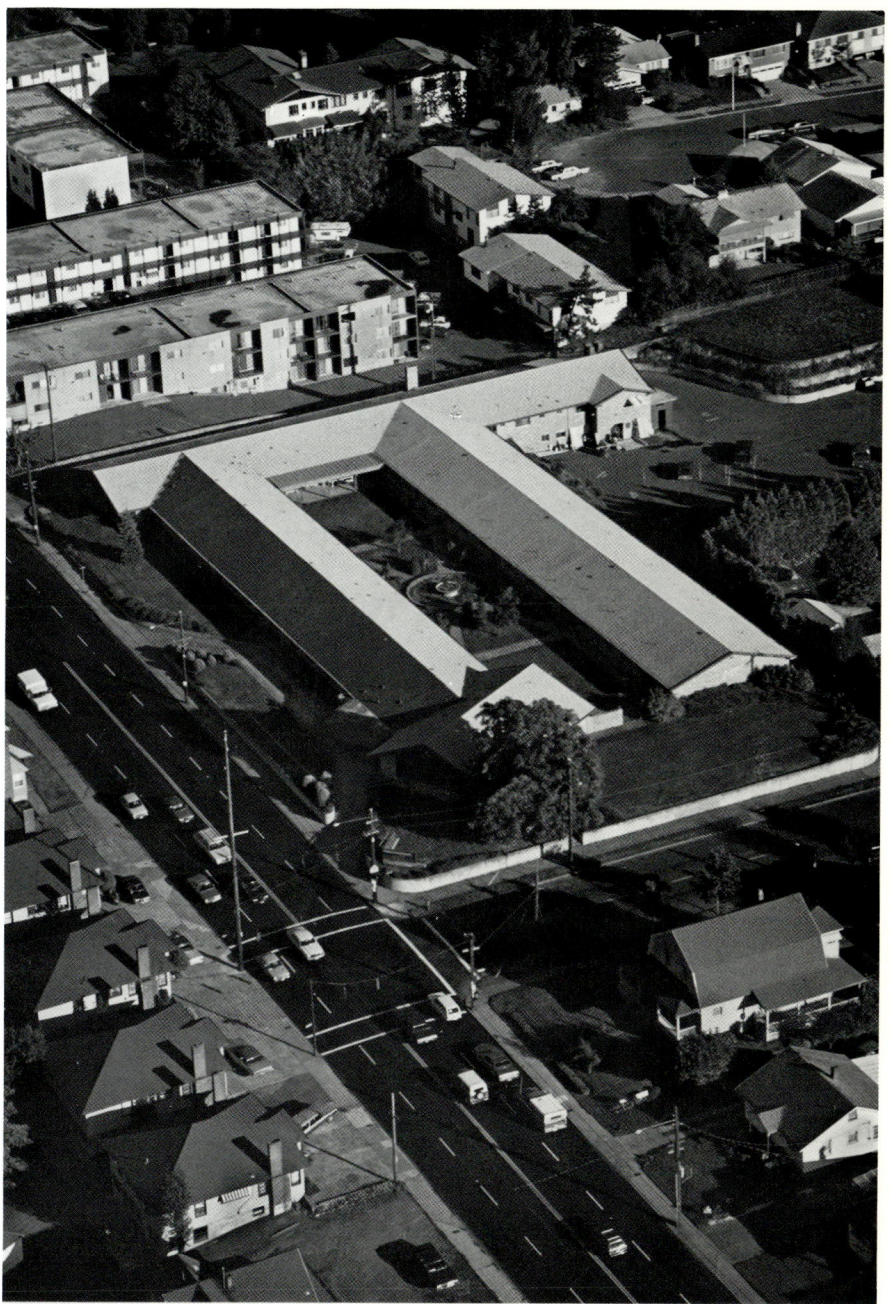

MIRIAM

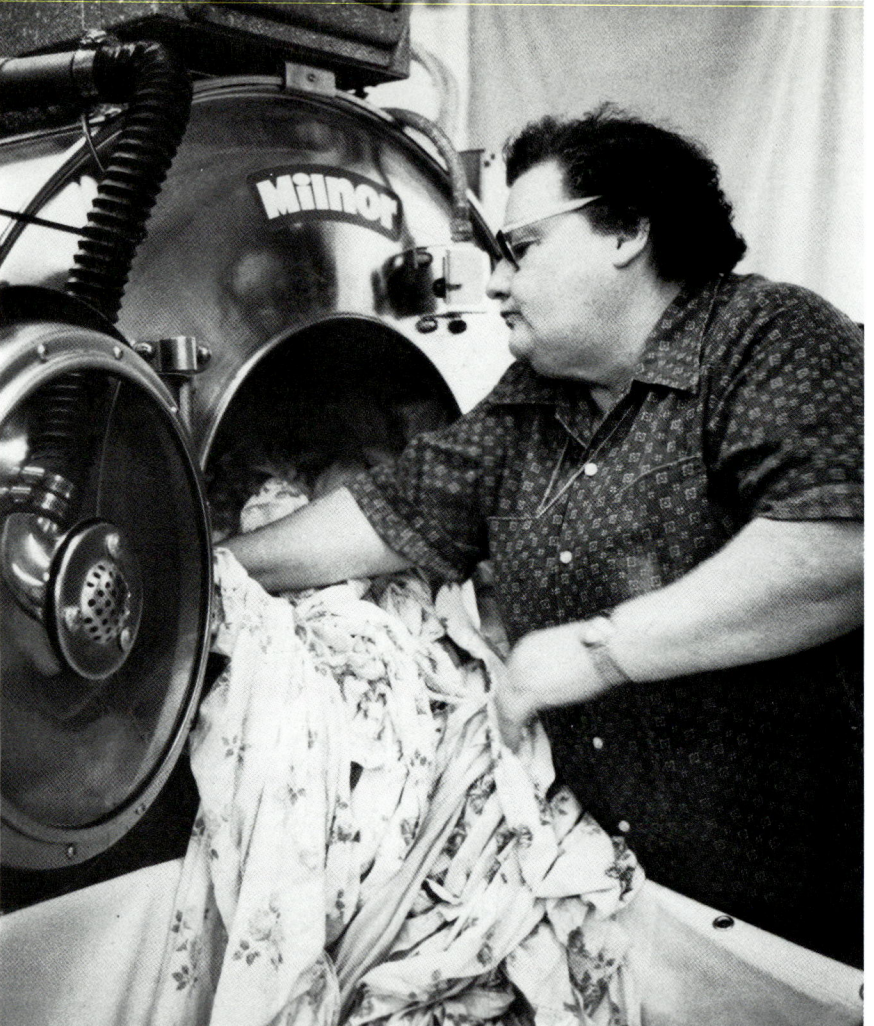

Until recently, Miriam was the supervisor of the laundry. Many of her employees had compiled poor work records as aides, janitors, or kitchen workers and were sent to the laundry as their last chance. Under Miriam's stern direction a number of them became reliable employees. Beneath her gruff exterior, she has a strong maternal sense; throughout the years she has taken several young men under her wing.

For over a year Miriam avoided us. Every time she saw us approaching her, she would dart around a corner. Finally, she consented. Hesitant at first, she gradually warmed up and talked into the early morning hours.

I've worked at this nursing home for more than twenty years, since it first opened in 1960. Back then it was a skilled nursing home facility; we'd get our patients right out of the hospital following surgery. We were called the American Convalescent Foundation. But we didn't have any competent help. Hips got broken, bed sores multiplied, so that status was taken away from us. When we first opened we had ten to twenty patients. Even so, we were always short of help, and I would dash upstairs after I finished my work with the laundry to help out.

I feel like I'm doing my part of the work in keeping the patients clean and dry. I enjoy it, and it's a challenge. The filthy linen comes down, and by the time I get done with it, it's back upstairs nice and clean and crisp. It's murder for those dear old souls to lay on rough sheets; their skin is paper thin. And if you've had a stroke and can't turn yourself over, you're miserable.

The patients come first. They're our bread and butter. I like to go home and feel that I've done something good. My day is complete. They got a man in here who doesn't know beans from bubblegum about laundry. He wants quantity, not quality, so he'll put four hundred pounds in a three hundred pound machine. And he'll stuff it all in the middle, instead of loading it side-to-side like you're supposed to. But we all have to work together . . . I'm not the boss here.

I will always remember that this nursing home has been good to me, gave me a job, tolerated me. Many times I've been written up for flappin' my lip, but I felt I was right. If I do hear something that needs to be reported, I tell it to the higher-ups. It's not right, for instance, when somebody working here calls a patient a bitch. If my mother was here and somebody called her a bitch, I'd knock 'em on their ass. And every patient is someone's mother, someone's father, or aunt or uncle. Every patient in here is somebody. The patient comes first.

I've seen administrators come and go. Some were not administrative material. I can't even remember all of them, they were here for so short a time. I do remember one who was only here for a couple of months. He was a former Navy lieutenant . . . goin' to clear all the dead wood out. His one accomplishment was to have the clocks changed to Navy time. But the one we have now, Ken, knows what he's doing. He's a former R.N., and if a patient looks bad he doesn't go down the hall and ignore it.

I'd like to see elderly people left in their homes longer. Let's educate people to go into elderly persons' homes, to cook for 'em and run the vacuum a little bit. Every day or every other day. If you can live in your home, have your things around you, you'll live longer, be happier. God knows, it's hard to give up your home. But if someone gets so they mess themselves up, can't feed themselves, then it's time for them to give up their home.

There are so many residents that linger year after year after year. What is the sense in that? They're a burden to themselves and those who have to take care of them. If you've lived long enough to see the handiwork of God—the ocean, the moon, the stars—you're lucky. Go to the ground where you belong, at peace. For the dead are all through and they ain't goin' to bite you. They're the lucky ones. Us poor devils, we've still got to be chosen.

—Miriam

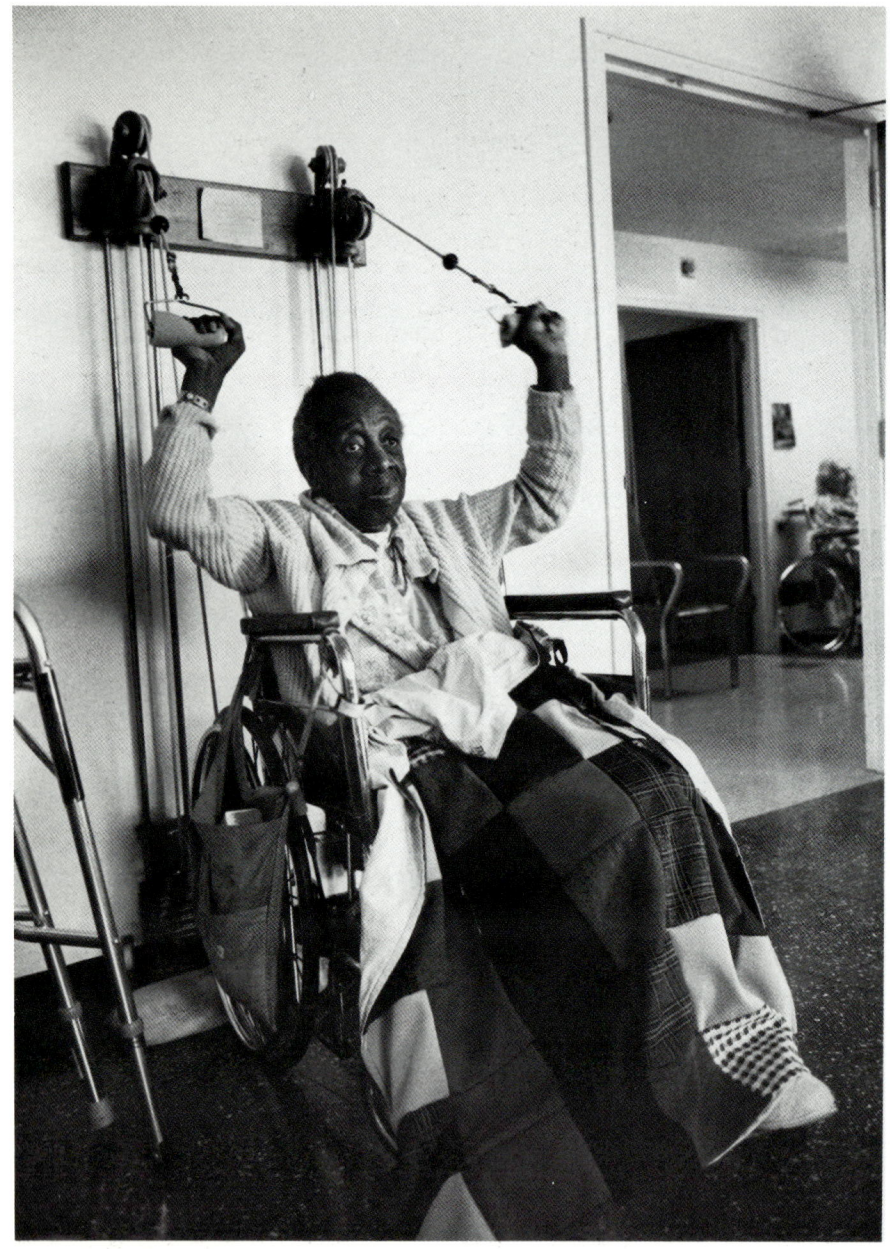

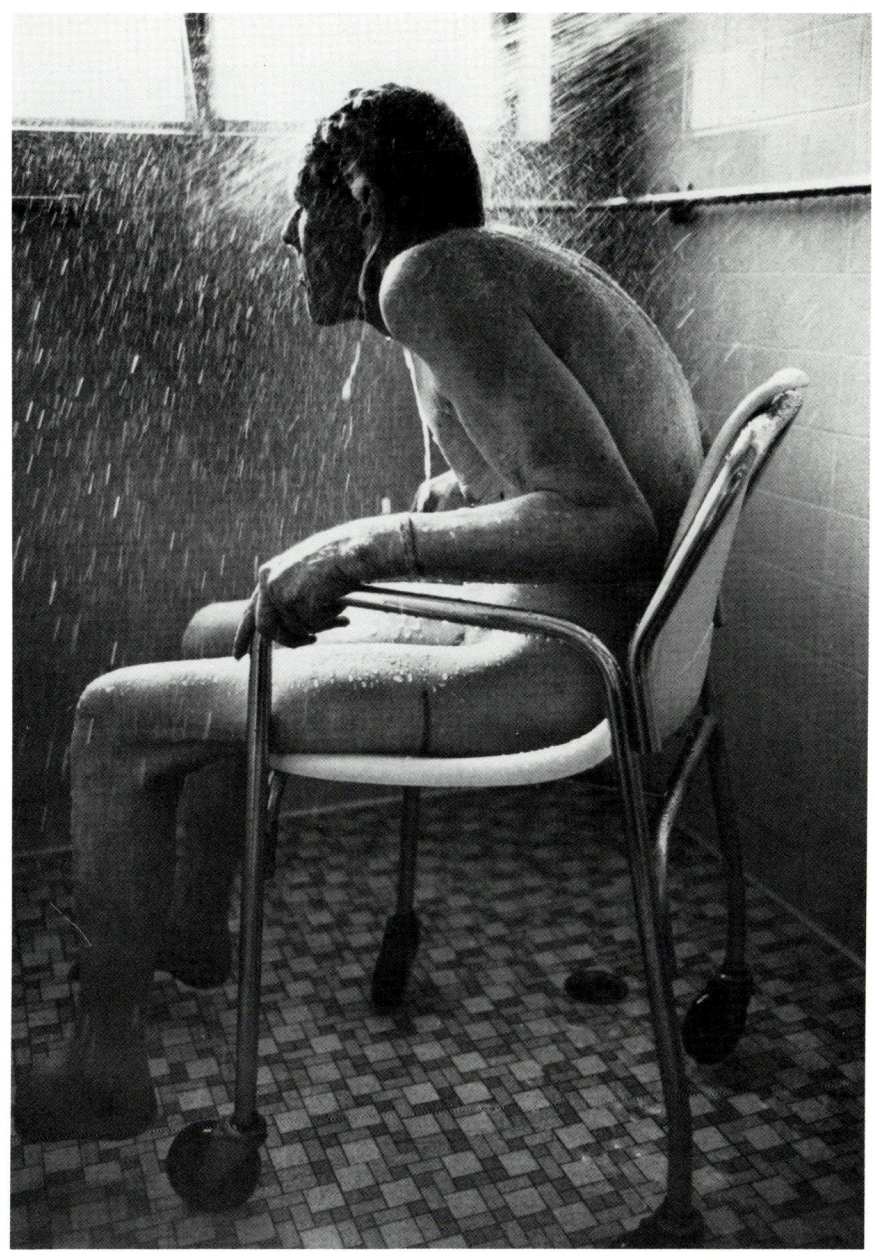

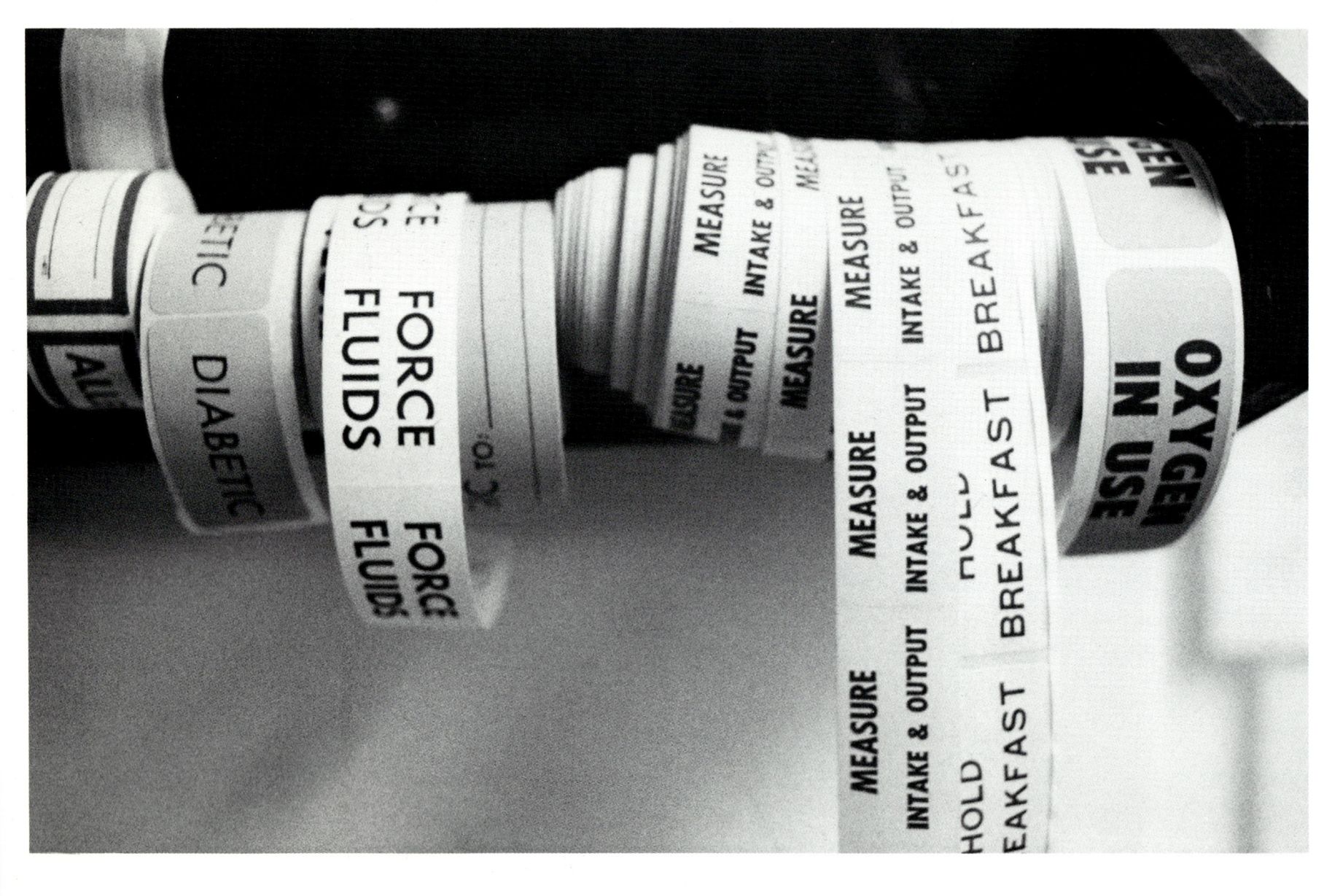

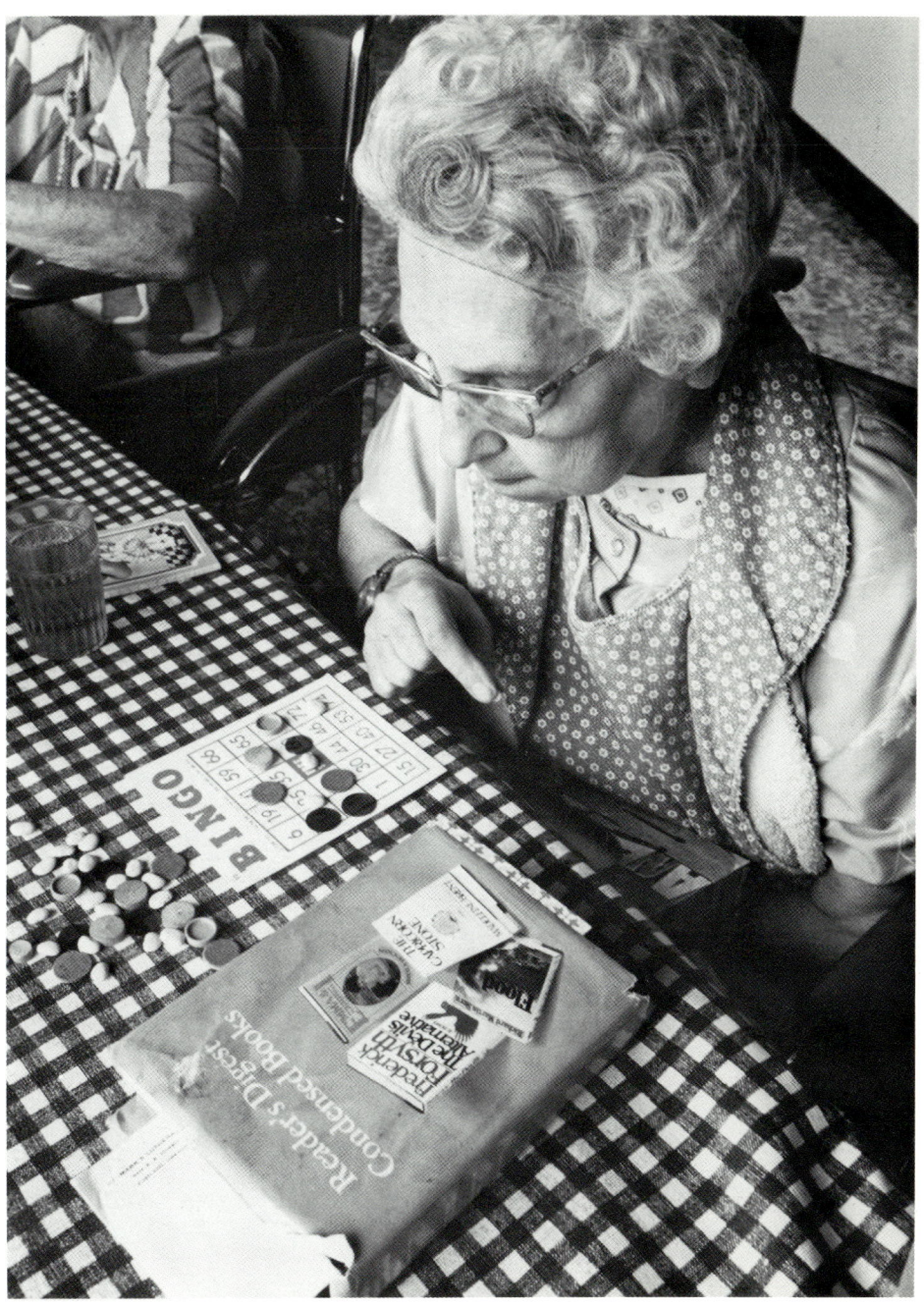

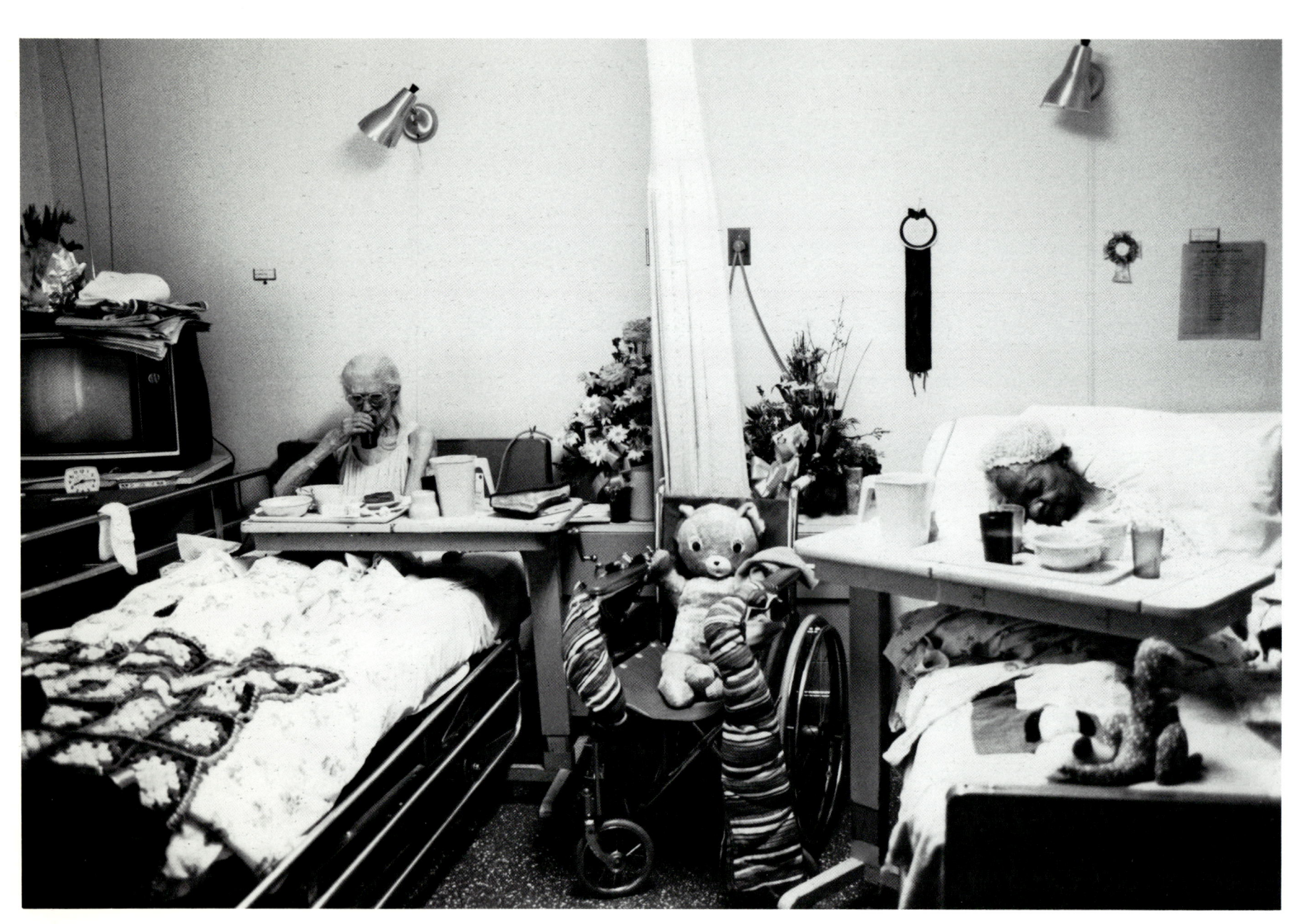

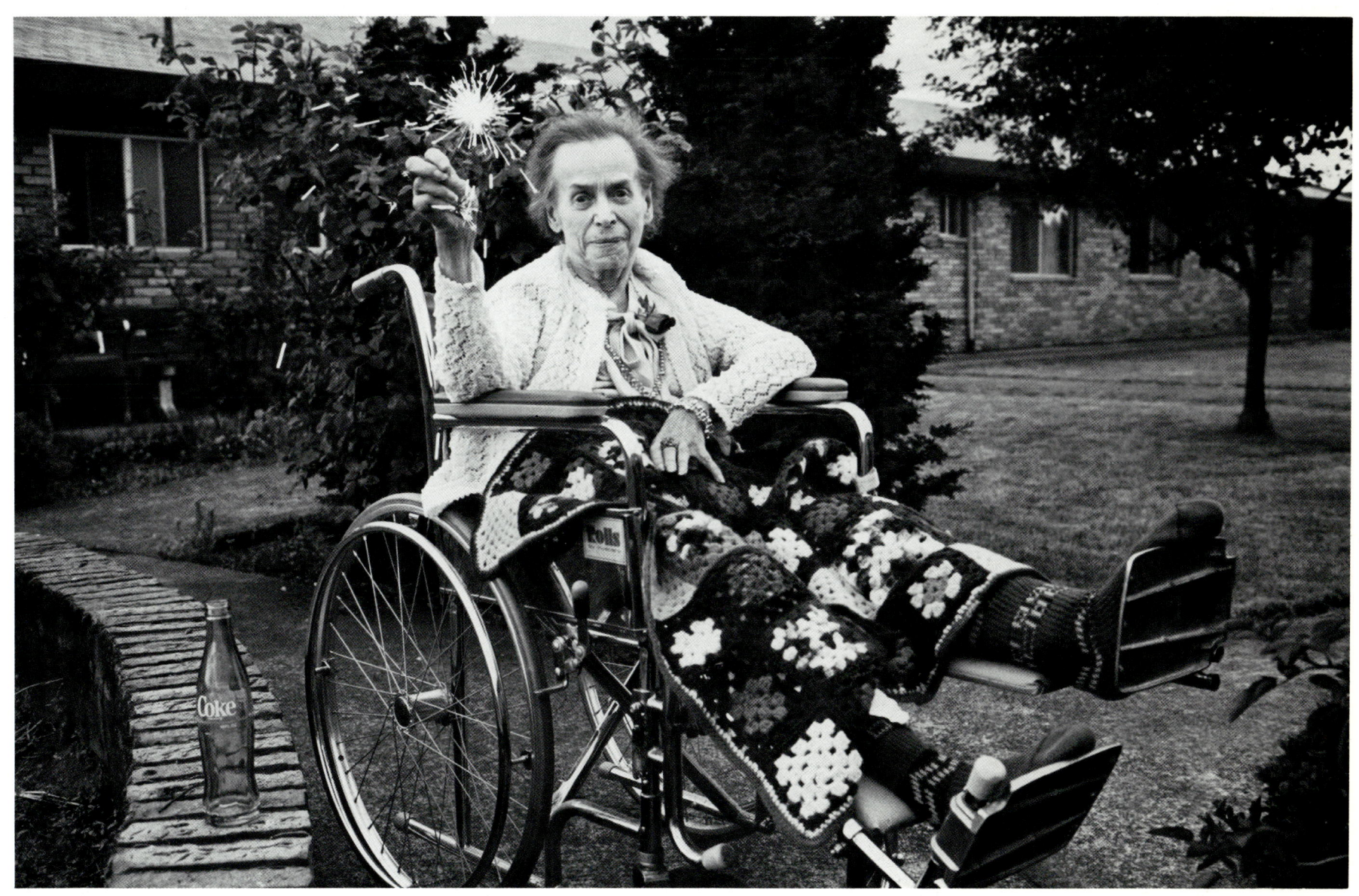

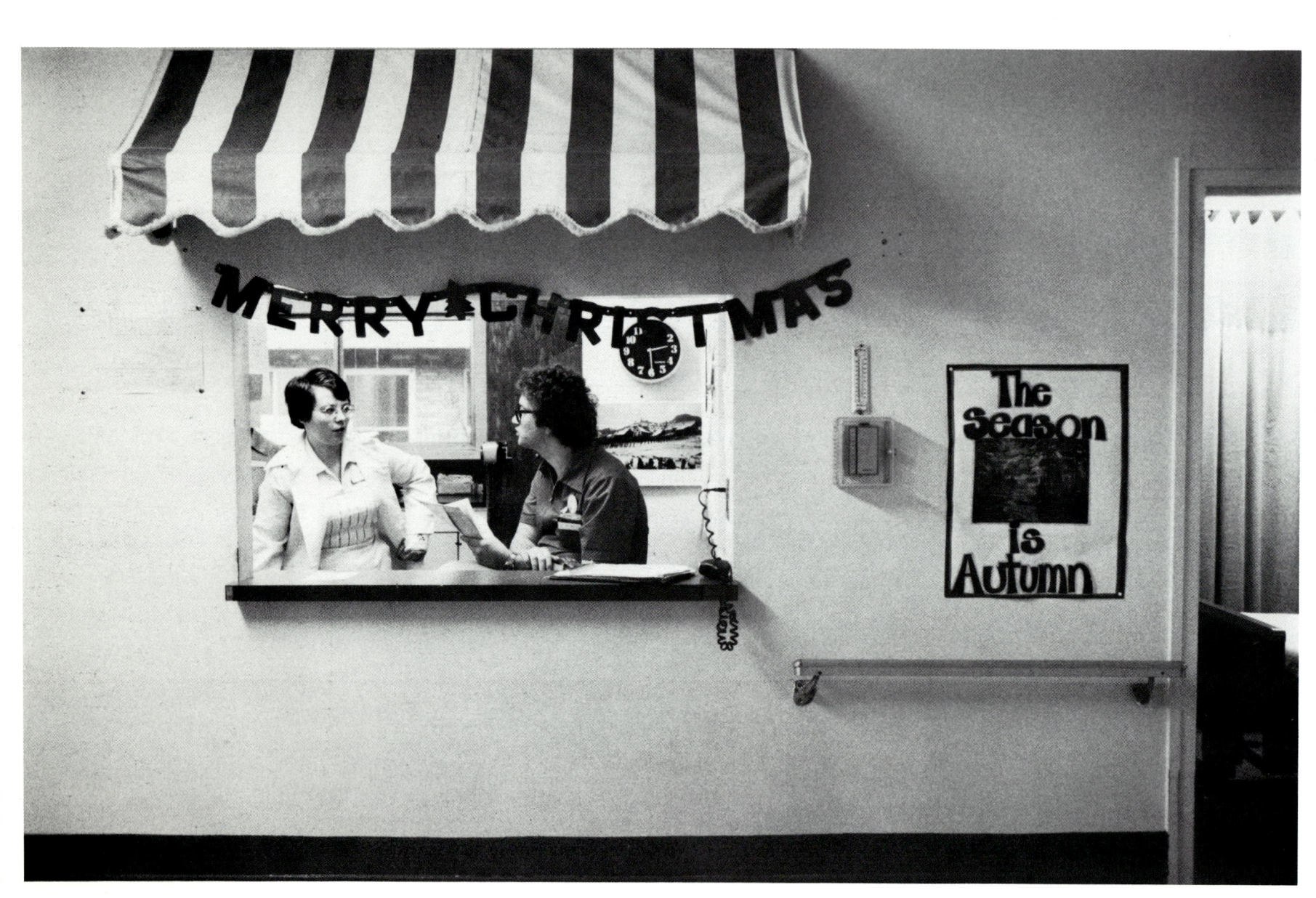

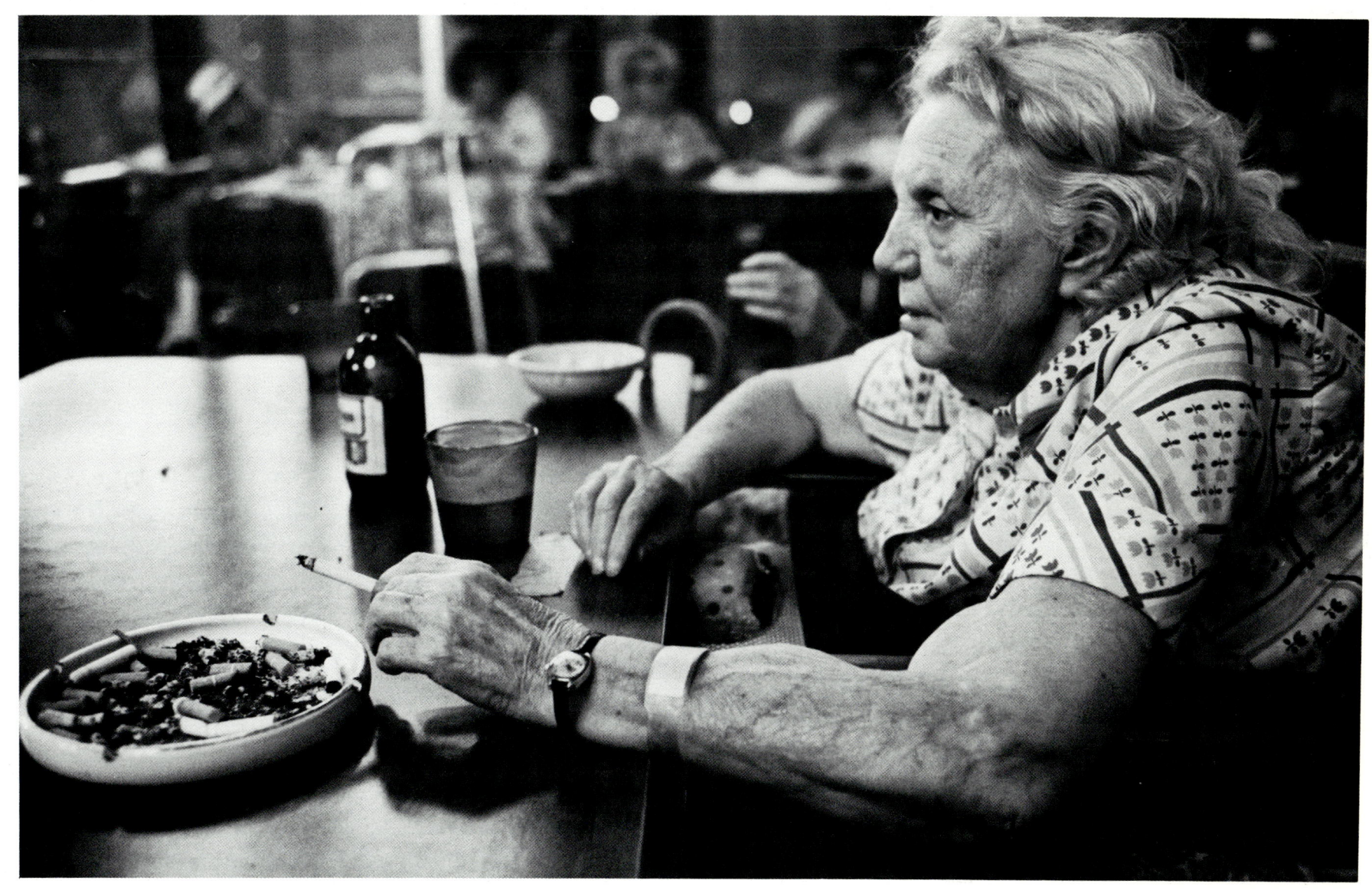

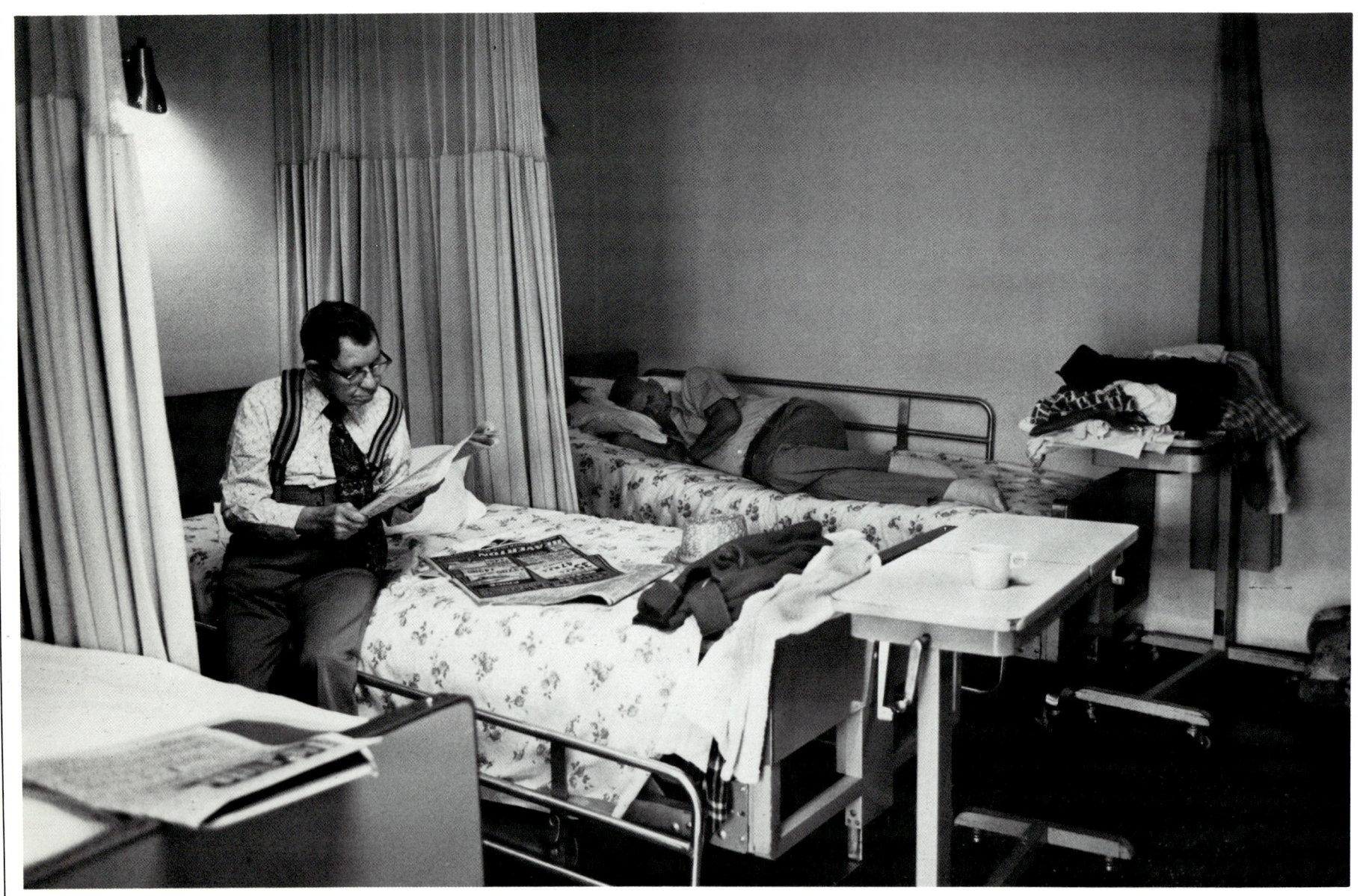

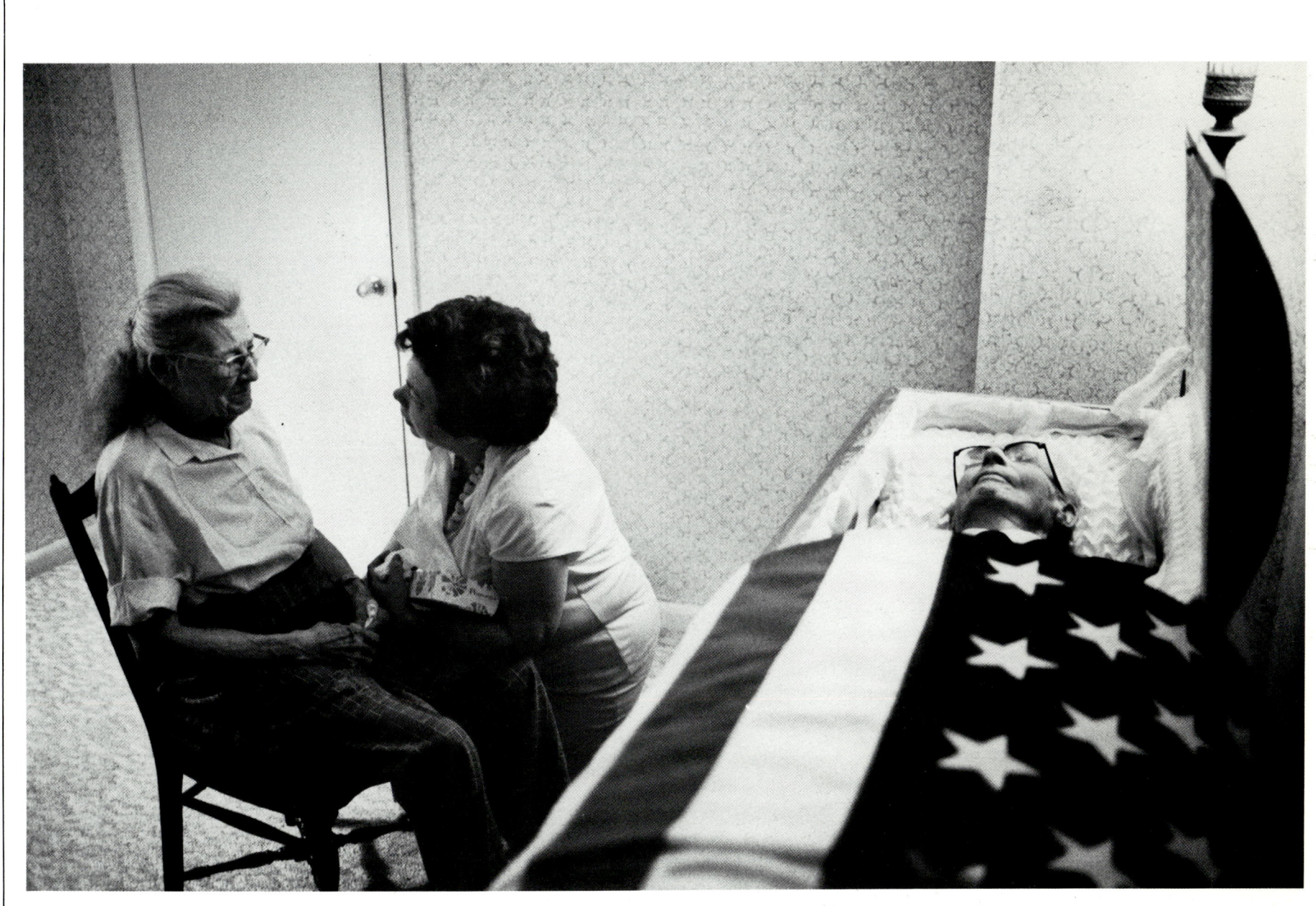

II. Links Forged and Broken

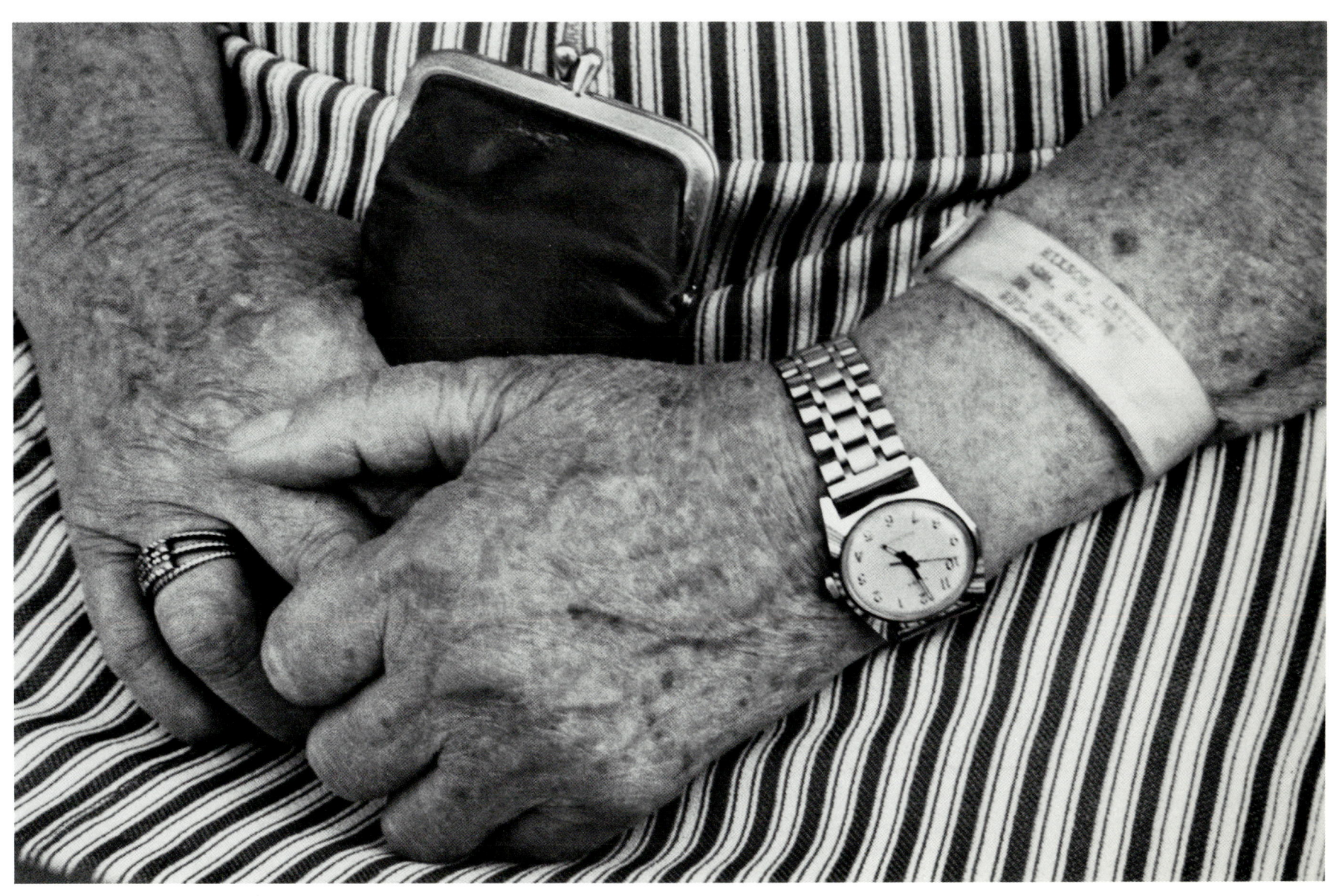

PAT AND HAZEL

Before Hazel was admitted to the nursing home, she lived with her daughter Pat. Pat ran a part-time secretarial service out of her home, and they managed to make do with a small income and Hazel's meager Social Security check. But Hazel's condition worsened, and Pat found that she could no longer care for her mother at home.

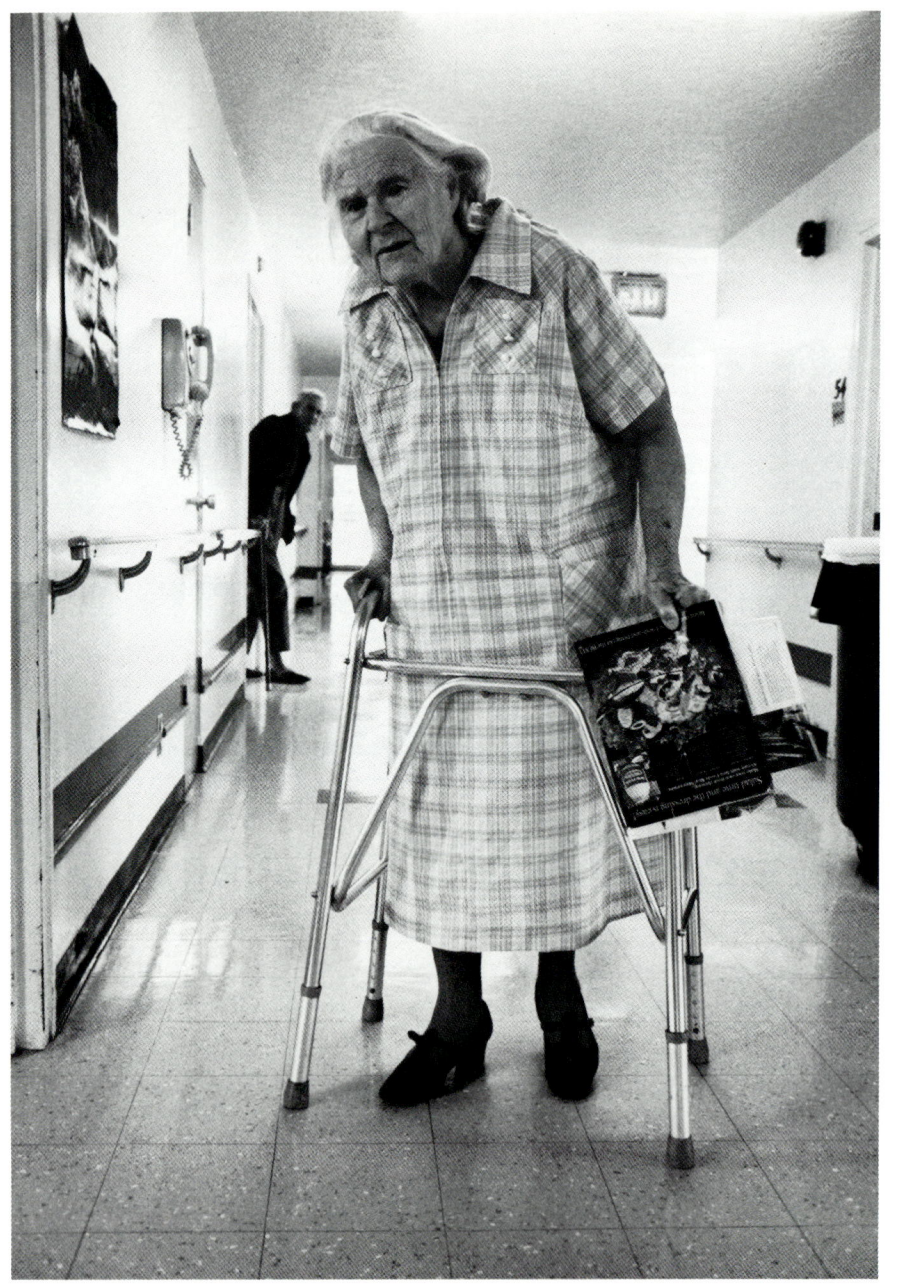

I had been taking care of my mother in my own home for the past two years. Occasionally she would become very depressed, knowing she was such a burden. How would you feel to have your daughter dressing and undressing you, and bathing you, and completely taking care of you? If it was an emergency you could put up with it for a while, but you couldn't put up with it for an indefinite period of time. I know I wouldn't want my daughter to have to do all that.

When I showed Mother the family album she often wouldn't recognize the members of the family. And when she did, she would mix them up with each other. She might mix my daughter up with me, or she would even mix me up with her mother. Half the time she talked about me being her mother. She would equate me with her mother, taking care of her.

Mother would do anything she could think of to get my attention. I would see to it that she was well cared for, that she had had her lunch, that she had gone to the bathroom, that she had everything she needed. I would get her some juice, and then I'd finally sit down to work. With the typewriter

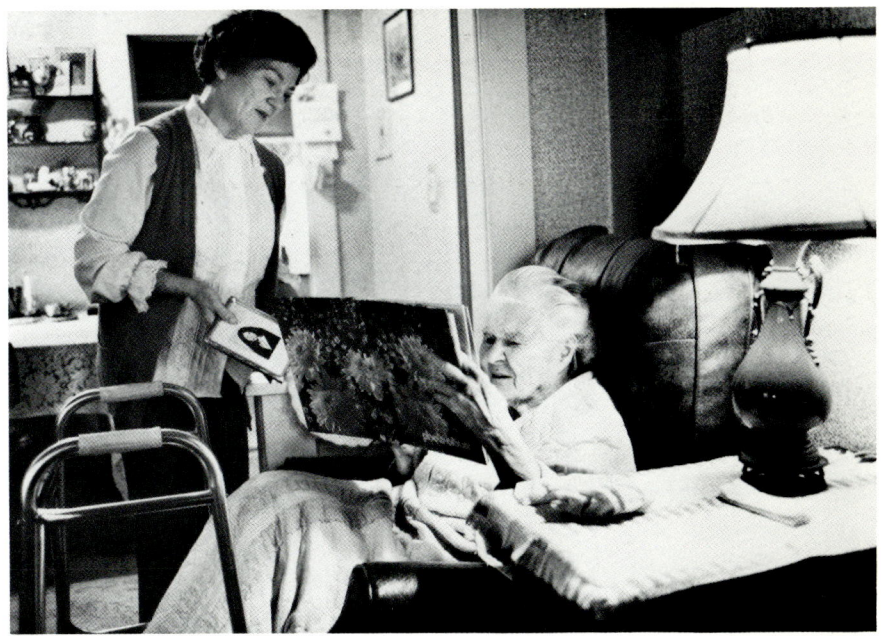

making a ghastly noise she'd call out, "Pat, where are you? What are you doing?" I knew that all she wanted was my attention, but I'd often have to turn the typewriter off for the day.

I finally realized that I couldn't take care of mother any longer. The doctors and everybody else said that she'd end up sitting there with me passed out and nobody to take care of her. If I had only had some help, but there are these damn asinine laws that allow the government to pay more money to keep a person in a nursing home than subsidize their staying at home. I didn't have the strength to lift her anymore. I couldn't get her moving. If I could have I wouldn't have needed to have sent her to a nursing home. But I was absolutely helpless. I couldn't do anything else.

I failed. It wasn't her that failed, it was me and my physical condition. I darn near didn't make it myself last year. I could have continued if I had been healthy. But I'm not the only one that failed. In a way the government and society failed, 'cause I couldn't get any help.

—Pat

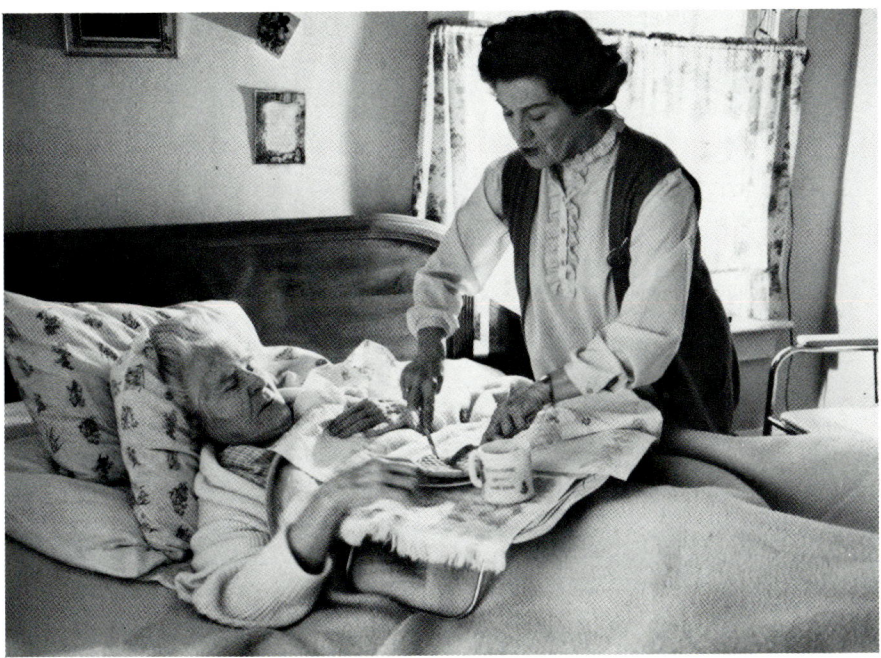

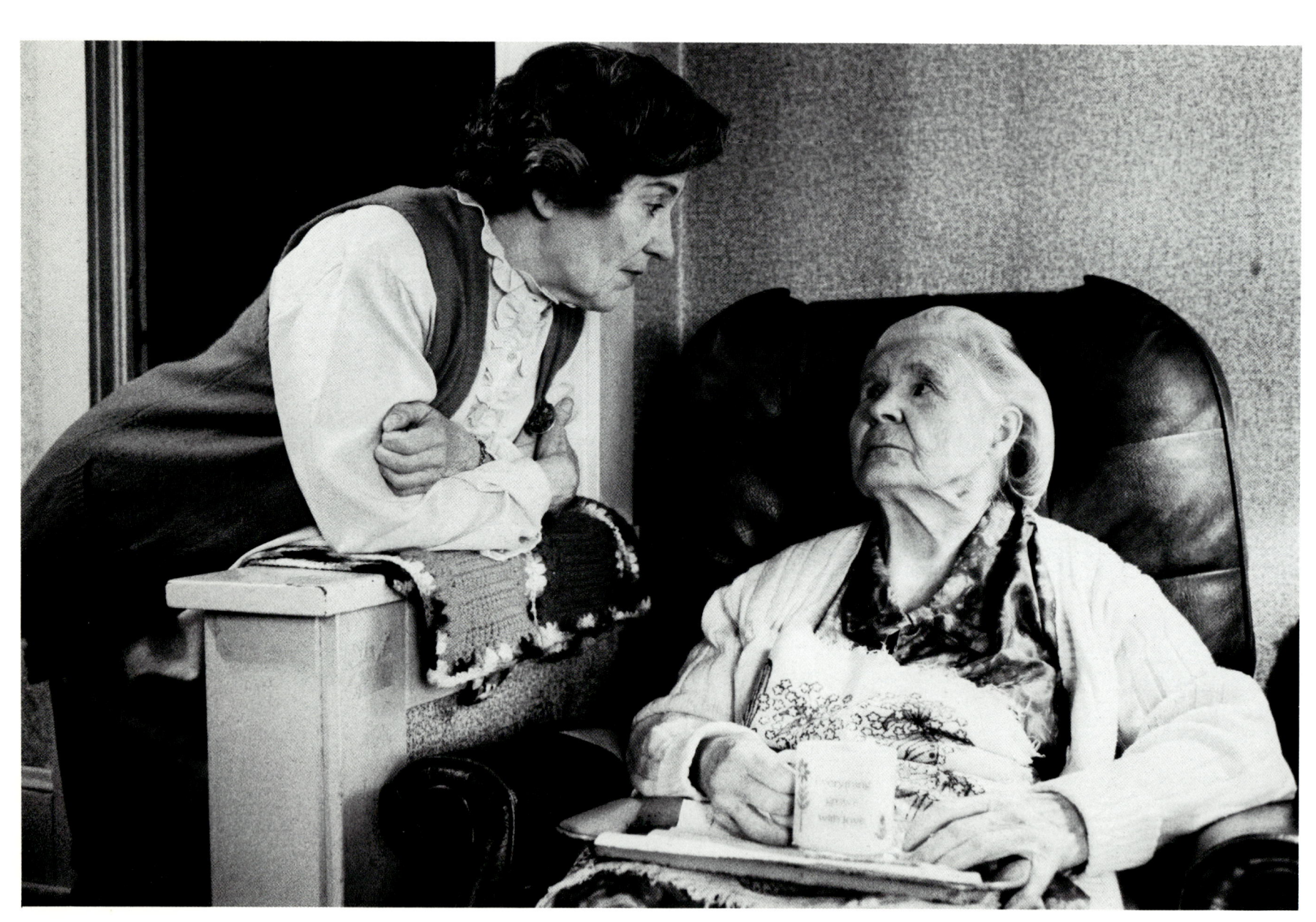

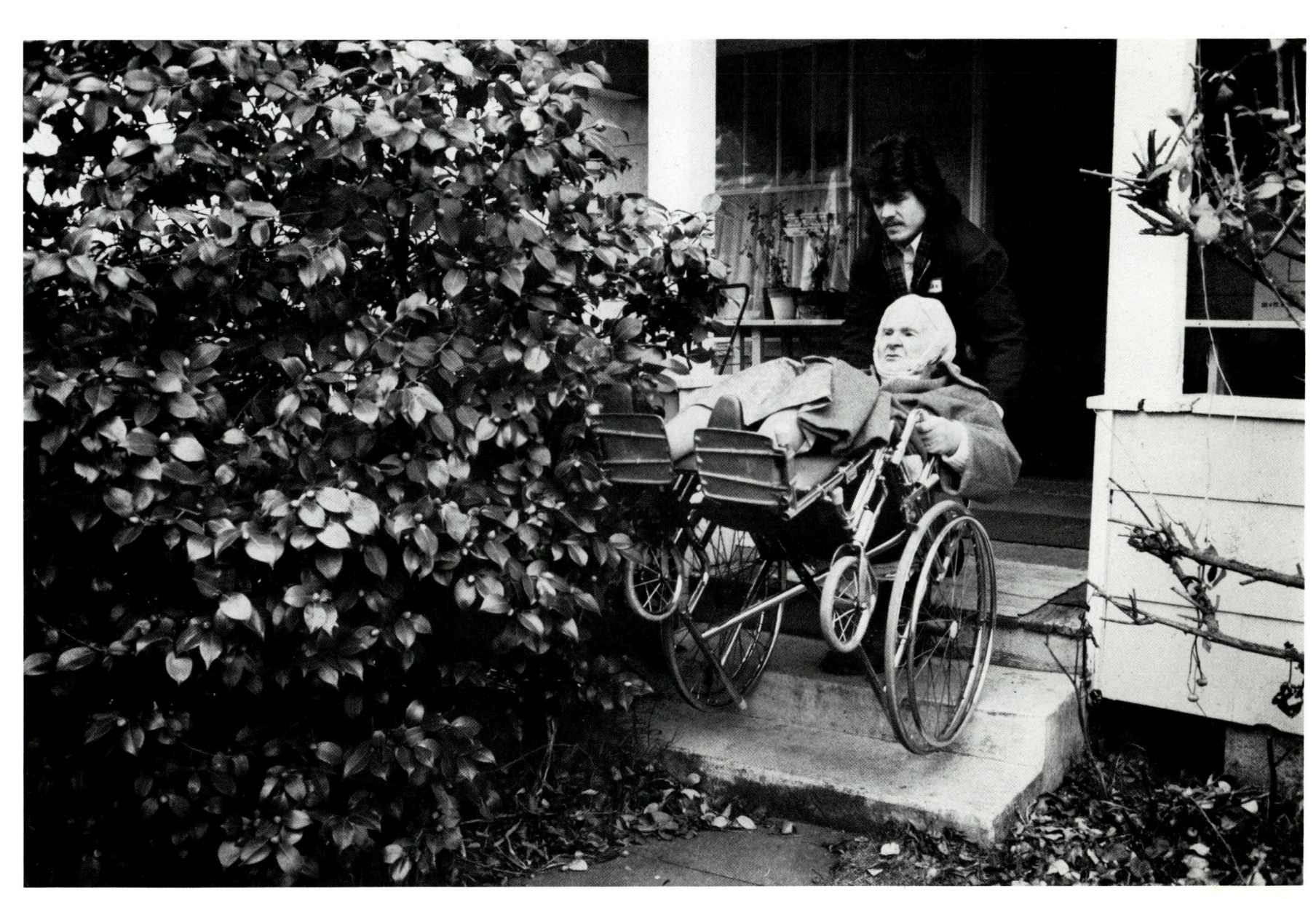

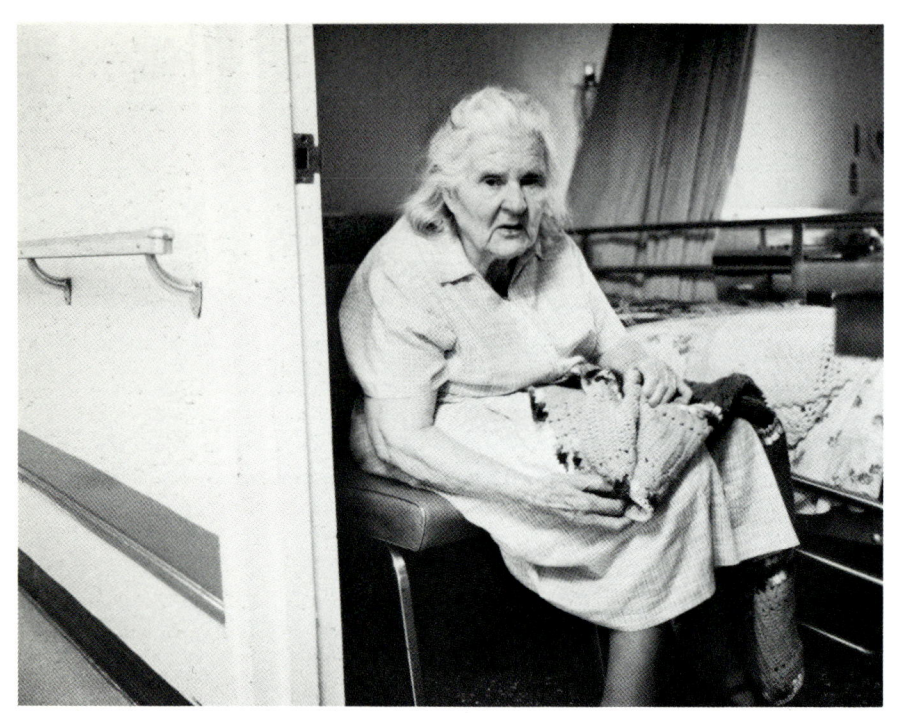

During her first month at the nursing home, Hazel rarely left her room, refusing to speak to anyone. Gradually her personality reemerged, and she became her talkative self. She enjoys kidding the staff and the residents, and her inquisitive nature sometimes leads her to rummage through other residents' drawers.

Pat visits regularly and has developed a warm and open relationship with the staff; she now realizes that she made the right decision. During most visits, Hazel does not fully recognize Pat, but occasionally she has clear days. Recently, Pat shared the family's plans for celebrating Hazel's ninetieth birthday. "That's fine," Hazel said, "just as long as you don't remind me of how old I am."

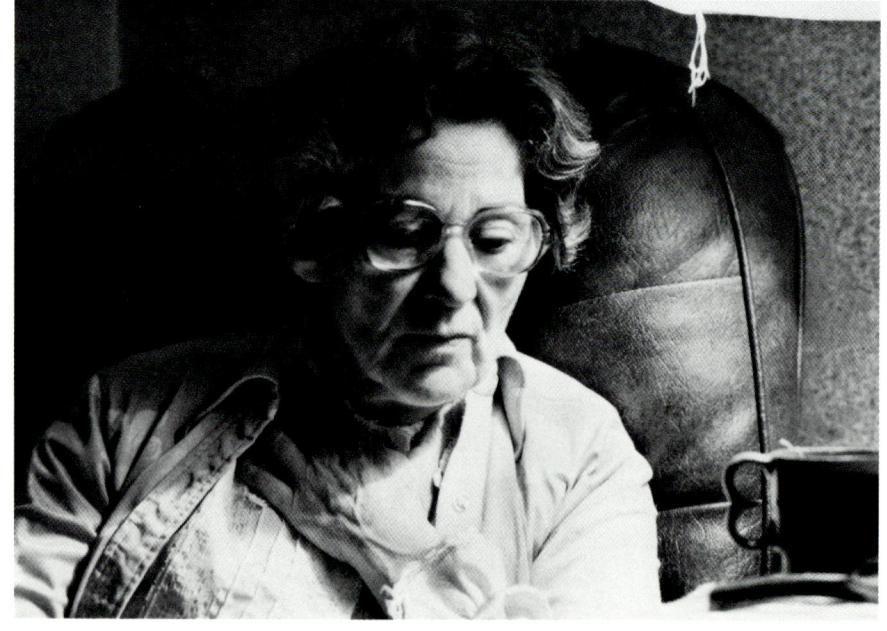

WILBUR AND CECIL

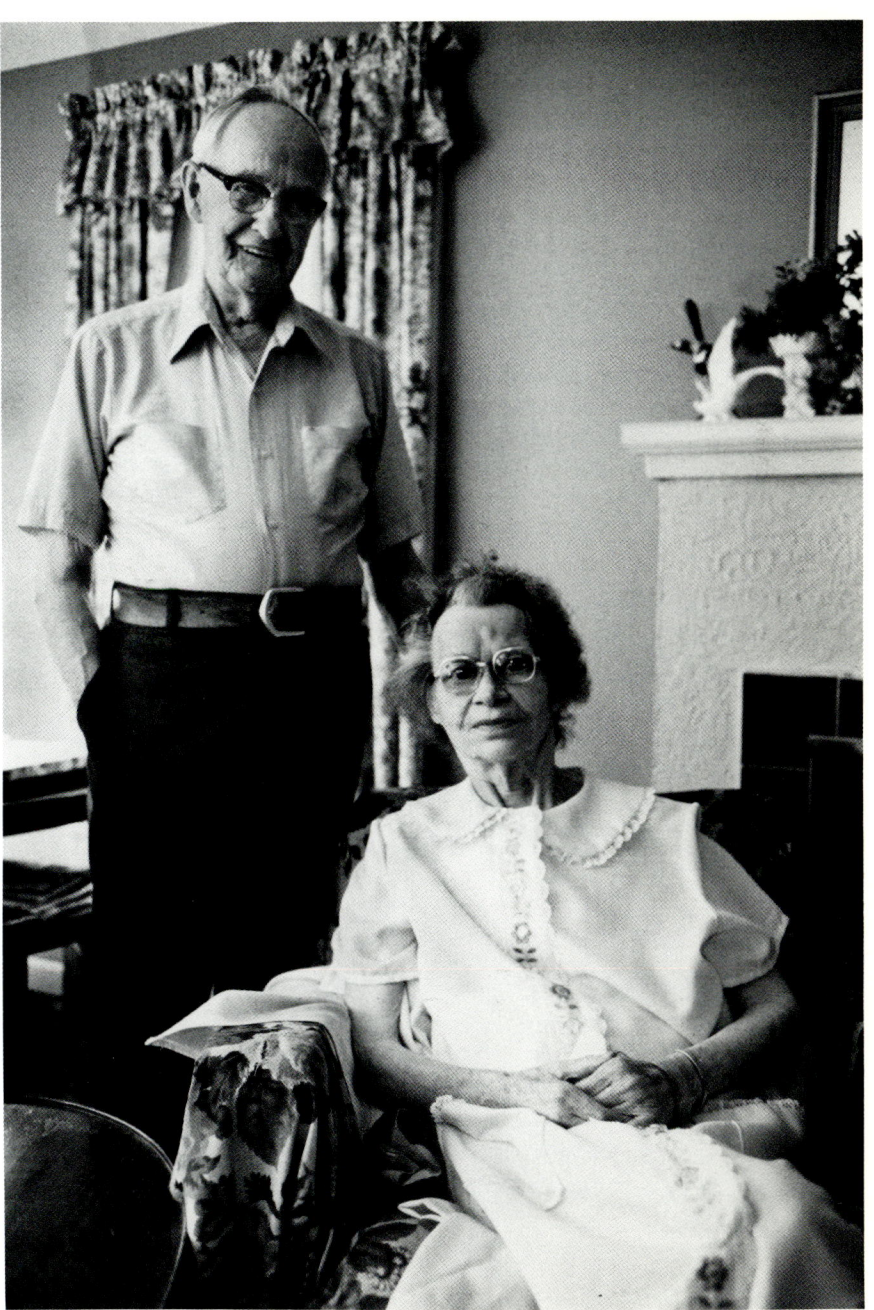

Friends from childhood in Pendleton, Oregon, Wilbur and Cecil married in 1942. For the last fifty years, Wilbur has worked as a rate clerk for a trucking company in Portland, but in 1975 he turned 82 and decided to begin working half time. Shortly after she married Wilbur, Cecil stopped working as a legal secretary in order to manage the household.

In the spring of 1976, Cecil had eye surgery for glaucoma, but the operation was unsuccessful and her vision continued to deteriorate. She became seriously depressed, and Wilbur had to assume full responsibility for the household cooking and cleaning. Three years later, Cecil came down with pneumonia and was sent to the hospital, where it was recommended that she be placed in a nursing home. Wilbur searched for several days until he found what he considered a suitable facility.

Cecil was very disoriented when she first arrived, but Wilbur made regular visits and with the help of the staff Cecil perked up. Eventually Wilbur arranged for Cecil to come home once a month for a weekend, with the hope that she might eventually return home for good.

If I can keep bringing my wife home on weekends, it does a lot for her morale. She wants to come home for good, and right now we're looking forward to it. But why bring her home for good if she's not ready? After a month or two she'd have to go back and maybe in worse shape. It wouldn't help her and it wouldn't help me. But I'm optimistic. That's one reason I've got to keep my health, 'cause if I didn't visit her at the nursing home every day that would set her back. I never miss a day—sometimes I will visit her two or three times a day. If there is any little problem I go over to comfort her.

It was seven months yesterday when I put my wife into a nursing home. It's pretty expensive there, but as long as I've got it, it's hers. I'll spend every dime I've got on it, and if we have to go on welfare, we'll do it.

I wish her mind would progress as fast as her body. When she first had cataract surgery over six years ago and started losing her eyesight, she developed a despondent attitude. I had to start putting a lot more effort into taking care of her at home. I would do things for her and she wouldn't respond. It was very hard to get her to exercise; for instance, either the sun was too bright or it was too cold. Maybe I made a mistake—maybe I was too good to her. I had a terrible time getting her to do anything.

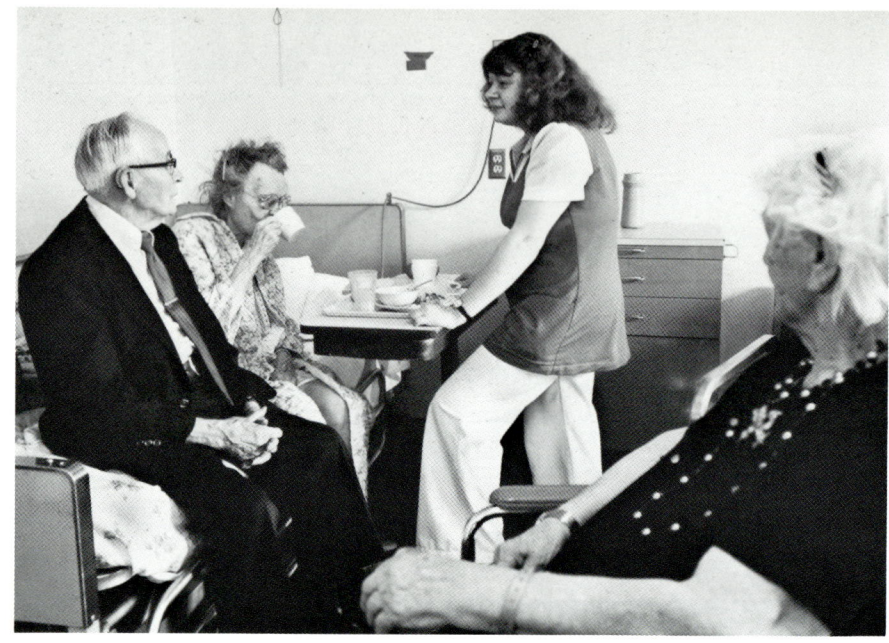

I made up my mind that what I couldn't get her to do they'd make her do in a nursing home. At the time I wasn't too happy about the thought of sending her someplace where they'd make her do something; now I can see that it was a wise thing to do.

It was rough when they first brought her over to the nursing home. She had the idea in her head that they were trying to hurt her. It took a lot of work on my part, their part, everyone's part, to get that out of her system. But we did! We won! She loves the girls now. They say that she is one of the easiest patients they have to take care of—that she does everything to try to make it easy for them.

The best investment I ever made was buying the nurses and aides candy and flowers every once in a while. Giving a girl a box of candy, a little flower—it just seems to lighten them up. You can see a real change right at the time you do it. I gave one little girl a box of candy and she just started to bawl and cry. She said that nobody had ever done anything like that for her in her life. She was just so thrilled. There wasn't a day she wouldn't come in and say, "Anything you want Cecil?" See what it did? And it didn't amount to much—maybe seventy-five to a hundred dollars. Every one of them, without exception, just lights up like a light when you do these little things for them. Wonderful investment!

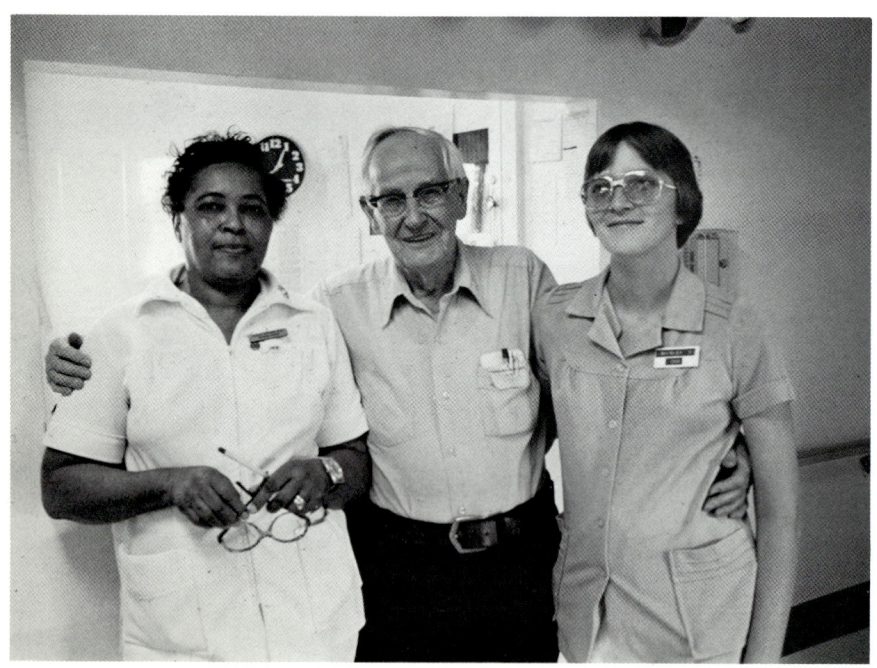

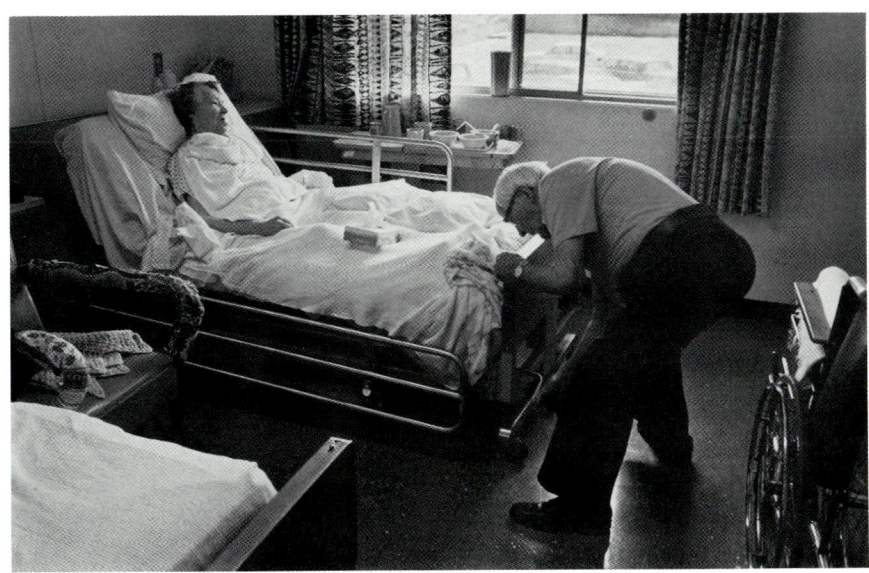

Wilbur's daily visits to his wife gave us the opportunity to become friends, and several times Rob and I offered our help in interceding for him when he was having problems with the nursing home. He listened, nodding his head politely, and invariably said, "Thank you boys, but I'll take care of it myself." As we found out, he was quite a formidable advocate for his wife—adept at using either the carrot or the stick. Both staff and residents look forward to Wilbur's daily visits: his presence invigorates the place.

Last weekend I went over to see Cecil and things were out of order—her room was a mess. At noon, when I came back to feed her, it was still a mess. They brought in her lunch and didn't even bother to empty her bedpan, which was lying on her bedside table. I got pretty mad, and when Monday came I really blew up at Ken, the administrator. I told him exactly what happened, and that I was thinking of pulling Cecil out of the home. Ken shook his head, saying that it was terrible, and he assured me that he would straighten it out. After that, Cecil's room was immaculate for a long time. They put forth a little bit of extra effort, to keep me from hollering. I'm paying almost twenty thousand a year, and I think that I'm entitled to complain. That's one thing I like about Ken—when I blow my cork he'll always say that I've got a holler coming.

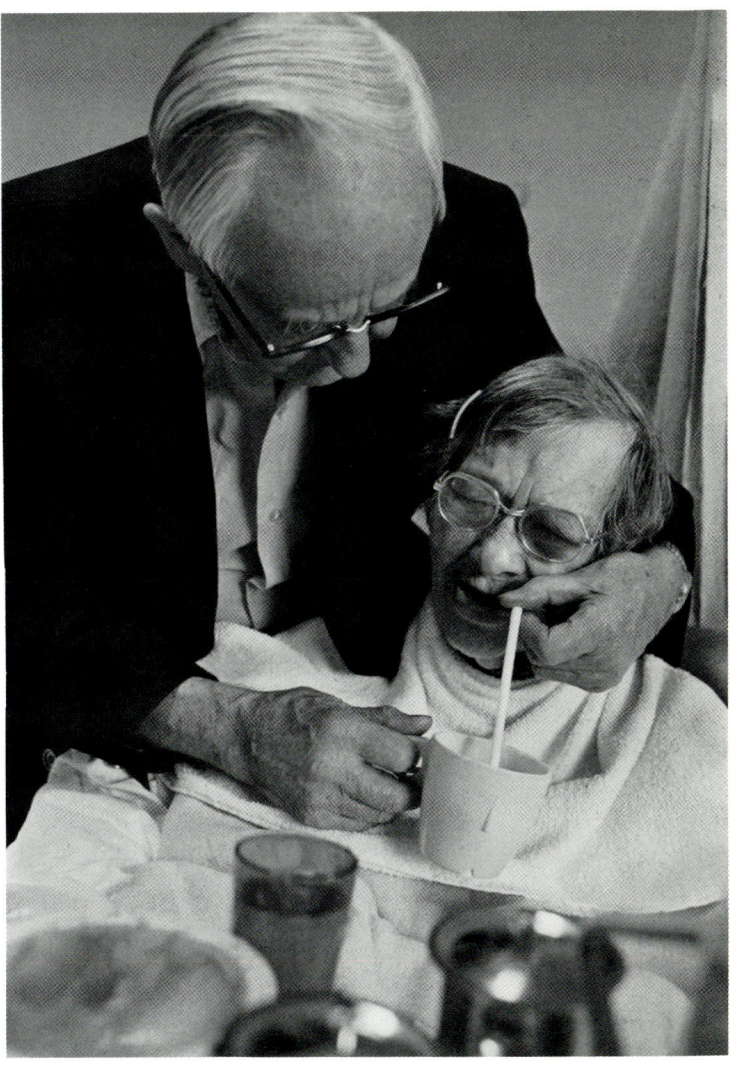

Cecil's getting worse. I asked Ken, "Is my wife deteriorating?" He said, "Yes, Wilbur," dropping his hands just like that.

I now spend an hour-and-a-half every noon feeding her. I think that she does eat better from me than she does from the girls. They just don't have the time; they have other patients. Yesterday I got 880 cc's of liquid into her. This is keeping her from dehydrating, you see. Today, I didn't do quite so well—only got 720 cc. But that's not bad; yesterday morning I see they only got 120 cc's into her.

It hasn't been too happy around home for me since Cecil went to the nursing home. It's been rough, awfully rough. The last two years have made an old man out of me—I'm not as active and alert as I used to be. But I try to keep busy and do quite a bit of reading, so my world doesn't revolve around the nursing home or being lonely.

If I saw Cecil improving every day, maybe I would have a more positive attitude, but she's only getting worse now. When I visit her, she doesn't carry on a conversation except, "I'm cold," or "I'm sleepy." That's it. She doesn't give me any support. It doesn't even enter her mind what this thing might be doing to me. But I know that she isn't doing this maliciously—it's just her condition.

I work very hard to keep myself from going senile. At work the other day, we were talking about old age and one of the boys said to me, "I don't know anyone as old as you who is still working." I'm holding up my end of the work, and they compliment me on what a good job I'm doing. But when I get to the point where I don't think I'm doing a good job, that's when I'll get out.

If anything happens to Cecil, I sometimes think I'll sell our home and move to the country where I can do some fishing. Then I tell myself, "Listen young fella, that might not be such a hot idea, 'cause I wouldn't know anybody." I would like to know what the future will bring regarding Cecil, but that's up to the Lord, not me. When He is ready to take Cecil, He'll take her.

—Wilbur

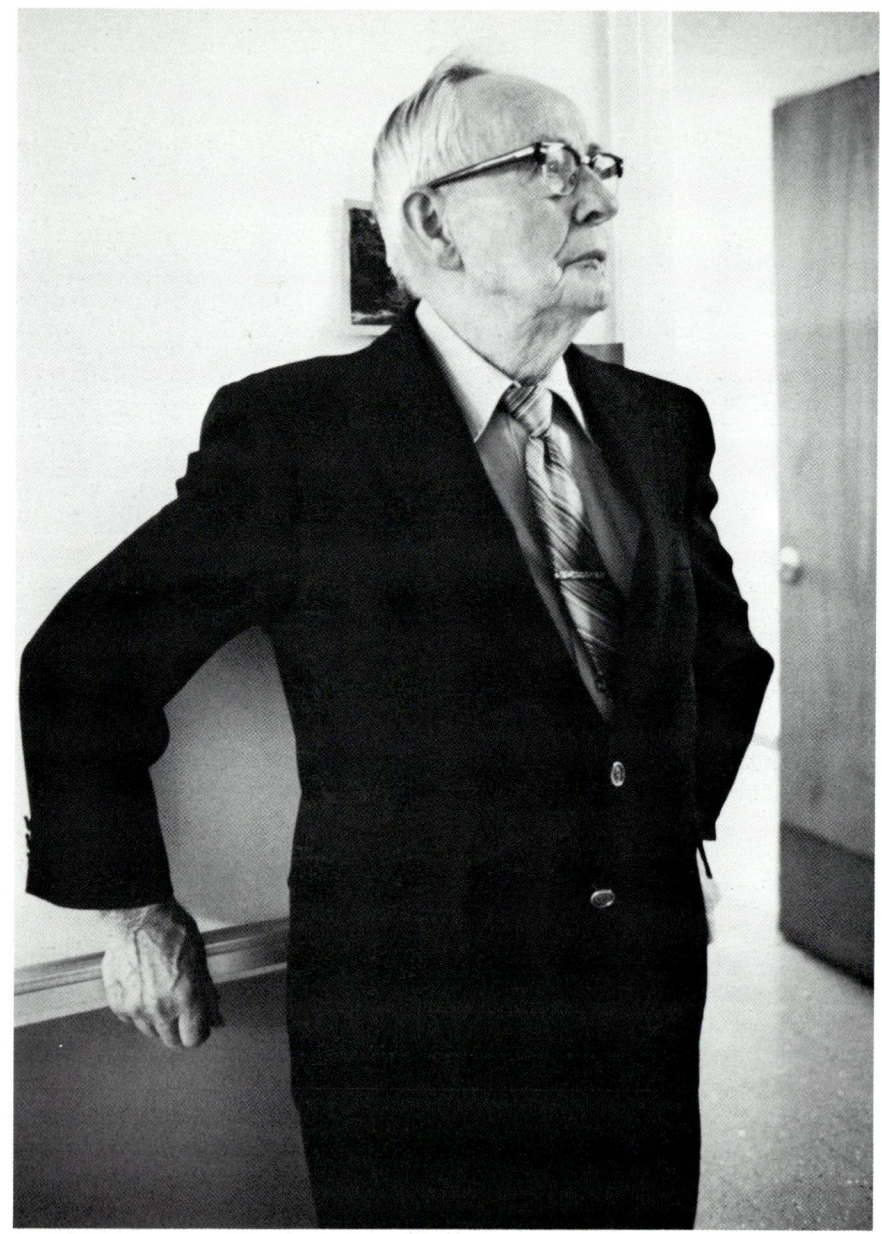

DONNABELLE AND GENEVIEVE

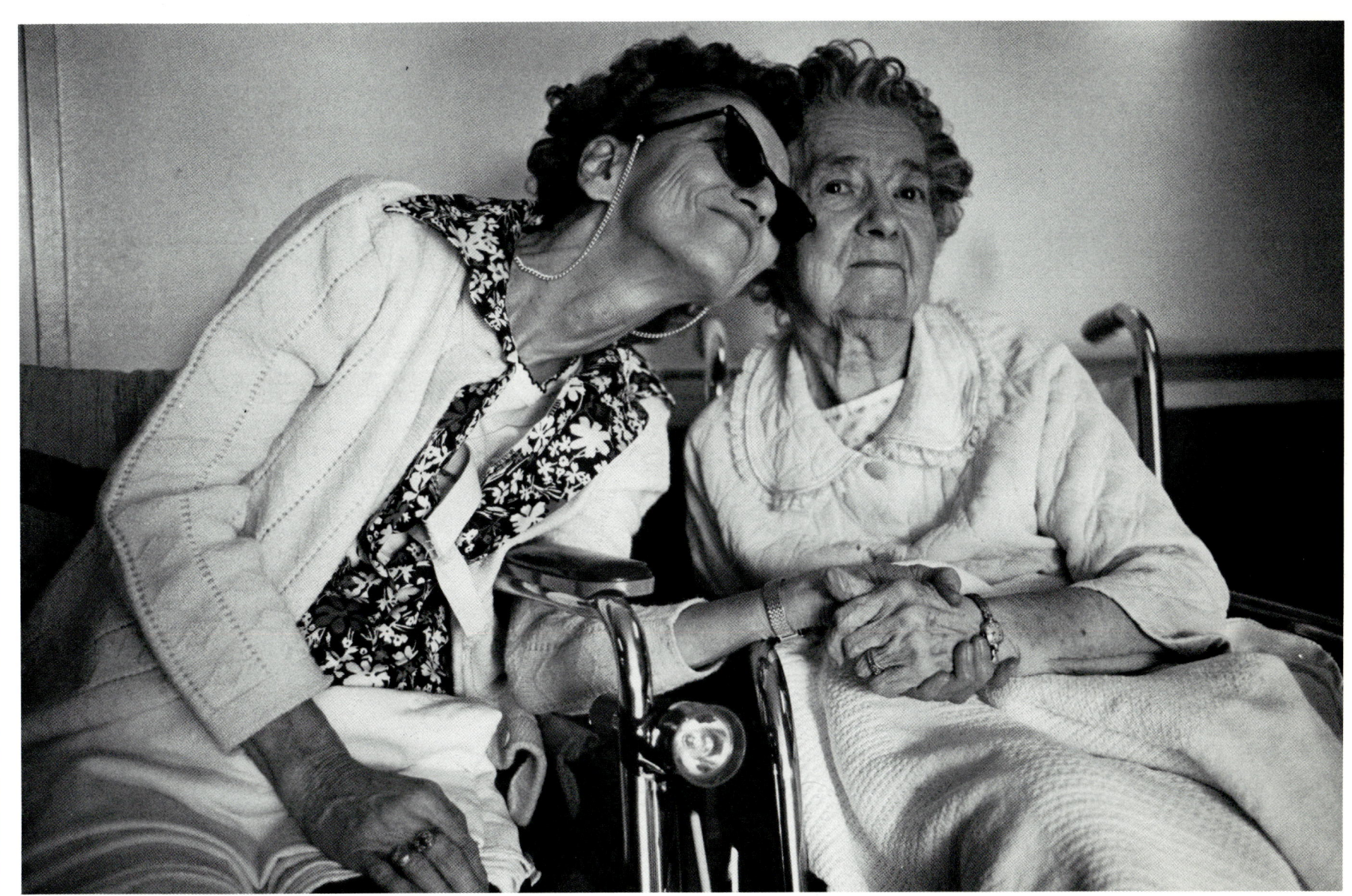

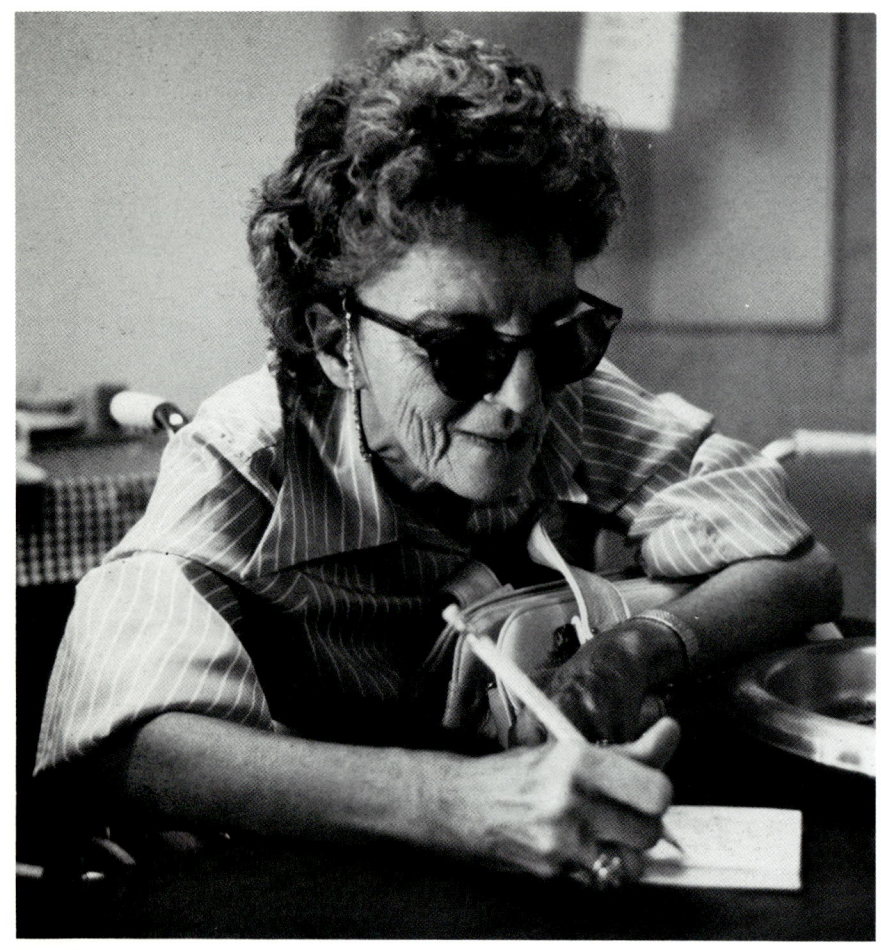

At 59, Donnabelle is much younger than the average resident, whose age is 83. Despite her physical condition, Donnabelle maintains a number of contacts with the outside. She regularly attends the multiple sclerosis meetings, goes on shopping trips, and goes for occasional outings with her ex-husband. At the nursing home she keeps busy working crossword puzzles, visiting with friends, exercising, and watching TV.

I got my MS over thirty years ago, just before I got married. My husband had a heart attack eleven years ago and he asked me to go to a nursing home while he recuperated, with the understanding that I could come home in a few months. But instead he filed for a divorce and here I am eleven years later. "You have a roof over your head, three squares a day, and all the care in the world," he told me. "What more could you ask for?" Then he convinced the family that I was riding on a gravy train.

When something important arises, my children still think I should consult their father. Like me going out with welfare yesterday to look at another nursing home; they thought I should call him and tell him about it. But I didn't. It's my business, not his. We're divorced and he doesn't pay any alimony, so why should I?

But we still see each other and he's pretty helpful. He does my laundry, buys me cigarettes, and even cuts my toenails. I'll call his office to remind him to bring his glasses 'cause he doesn't see too well and I don't want him to cut off my toes.

It really hurt my feelings when he divorced me. I just didn't think he would do that to me. I wouldn't do it to him. It says right in the marriage vows, "For better or worse, through sickness and health, through richer or poorer," at least it did back then. Yet he could go out tomorrow and rob a bank or kill somebody, and I would still love him. Not in a romantic way—it's been too long. He says he still loves me, but I think he loves the way I was in the past. Not the way I am now. It still hurts. It will always hurt.

—Donnabelle

Donnabelle's mother had been in another nursing home one hundred miles away. For over a year Donnabelle waged a campaign to have Genevieve transferred. She hired a lawyer at her own expense and wrote many letters to the Welfare Department. Her persistence paid off: she was given legal guardianship of her mother and Genevieve was finally moved.

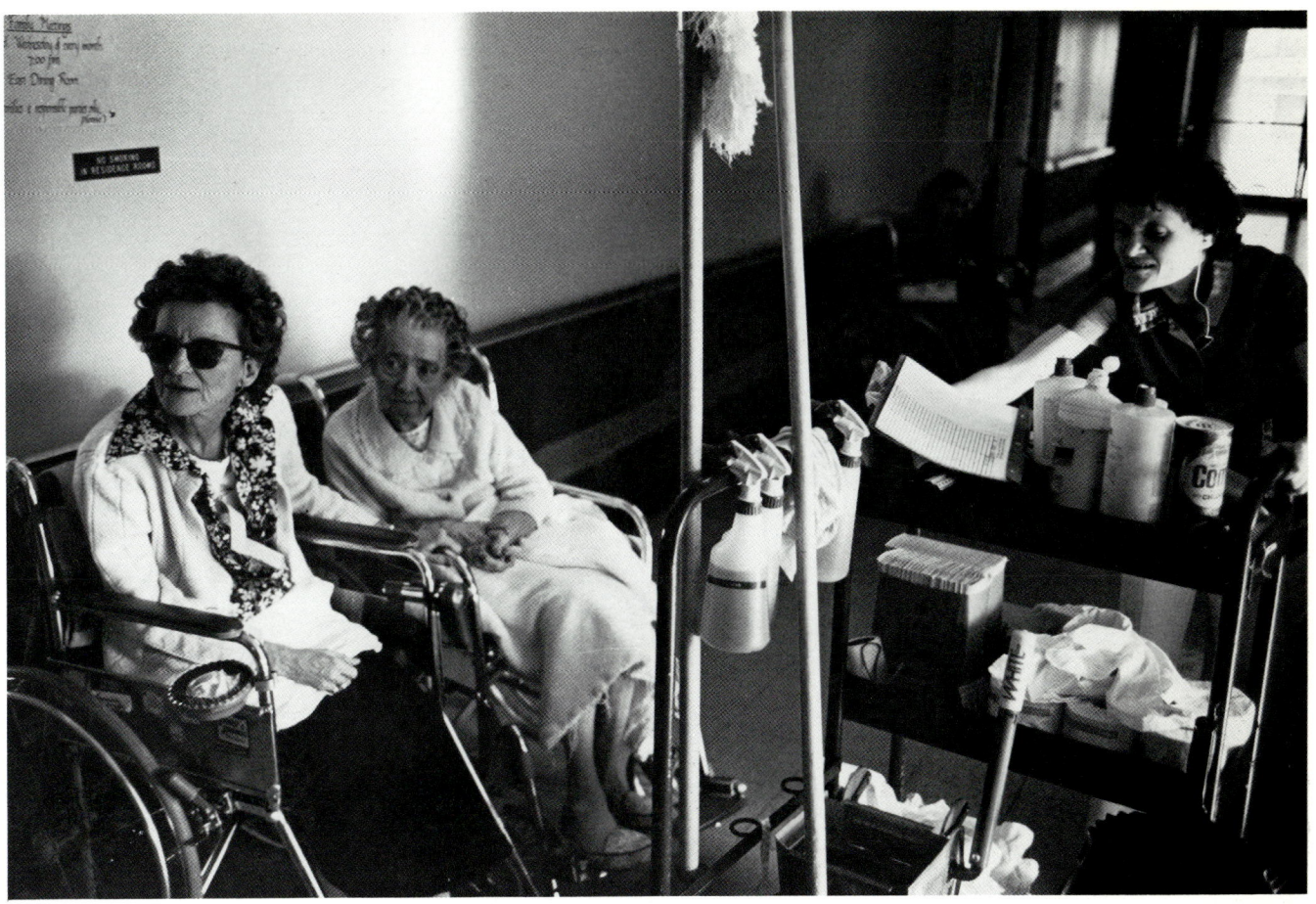

Mom moved in last year around Christmas time. I had her transferred here from another nursing home, so now I can help take care of her. She had a massive stroke about ten years ago. Though Mom is pretty alert for her condition, we don't know how fully she understands.

It hurts to see Mom like this; she can't carry on an intelligent conversation, she can't comb her hair, she can't put make-up on, she can't do anything for herself.

I take care of her: clean her wheelchair; look through her clothes to make sure that she has got everything that she needs. I even take care of her bills. If something is wrong over on her hall, all she does is say that she's going to tell Donna. That seems to do the trick. If there is anything wrong, I'll go to the administrator and fight her battles for her.

Mom gave to me when I couldn't give, so now I return the favor. Sometimes I am not well enough to do anything for either one of us. Then things just lay dormant for awhile until I'm up again, because I don't have anyone else that I can depend on. She doesn't either. Her sisters have told me as much.

I never realized how stubborn Mom was until she moved in here. If she doesn't want to eat or walk, she won't. Finally I told the nurses, "Don't ask her, make her do it." She never showed this stubbornness when we were kids. She was very dependent on my father then. He bought the furniture, the curtains, the food, and even bought her clothes. Mom never went out of the house except to visit a neighbor—that's as far as she got. Dad was the bigshot in our house. Now I'm taking over where he left off.

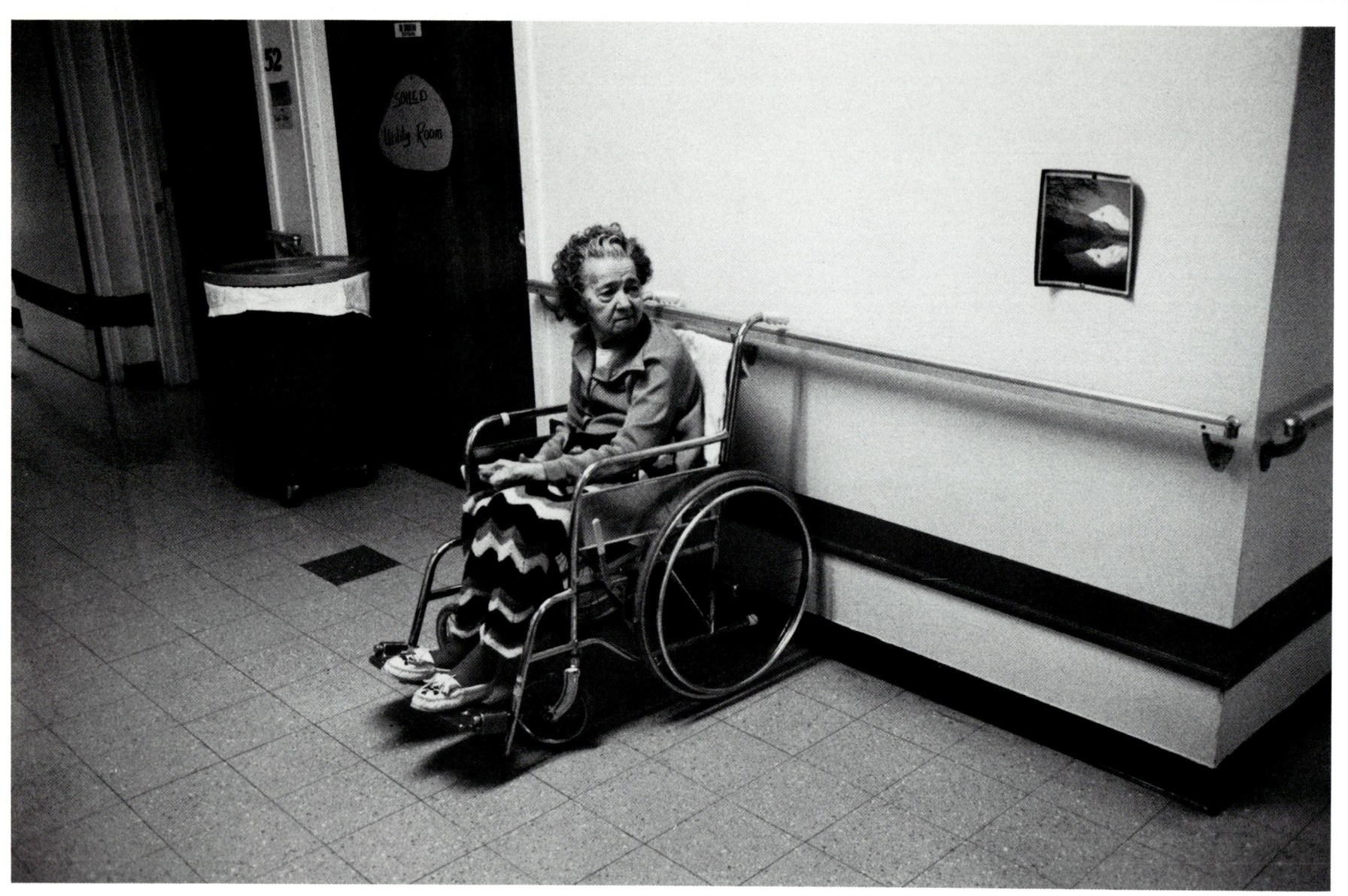

Mom needs a sense of security. For some reason that spot—between her room and the utility room door—seems to give her a sense of security like home did. That's her home—that one spot—and she likes to sit there to make sure that the darn utility door is closed. If it is open one little crack, she will close it. That door has always got to be closed.

—Donnabelle

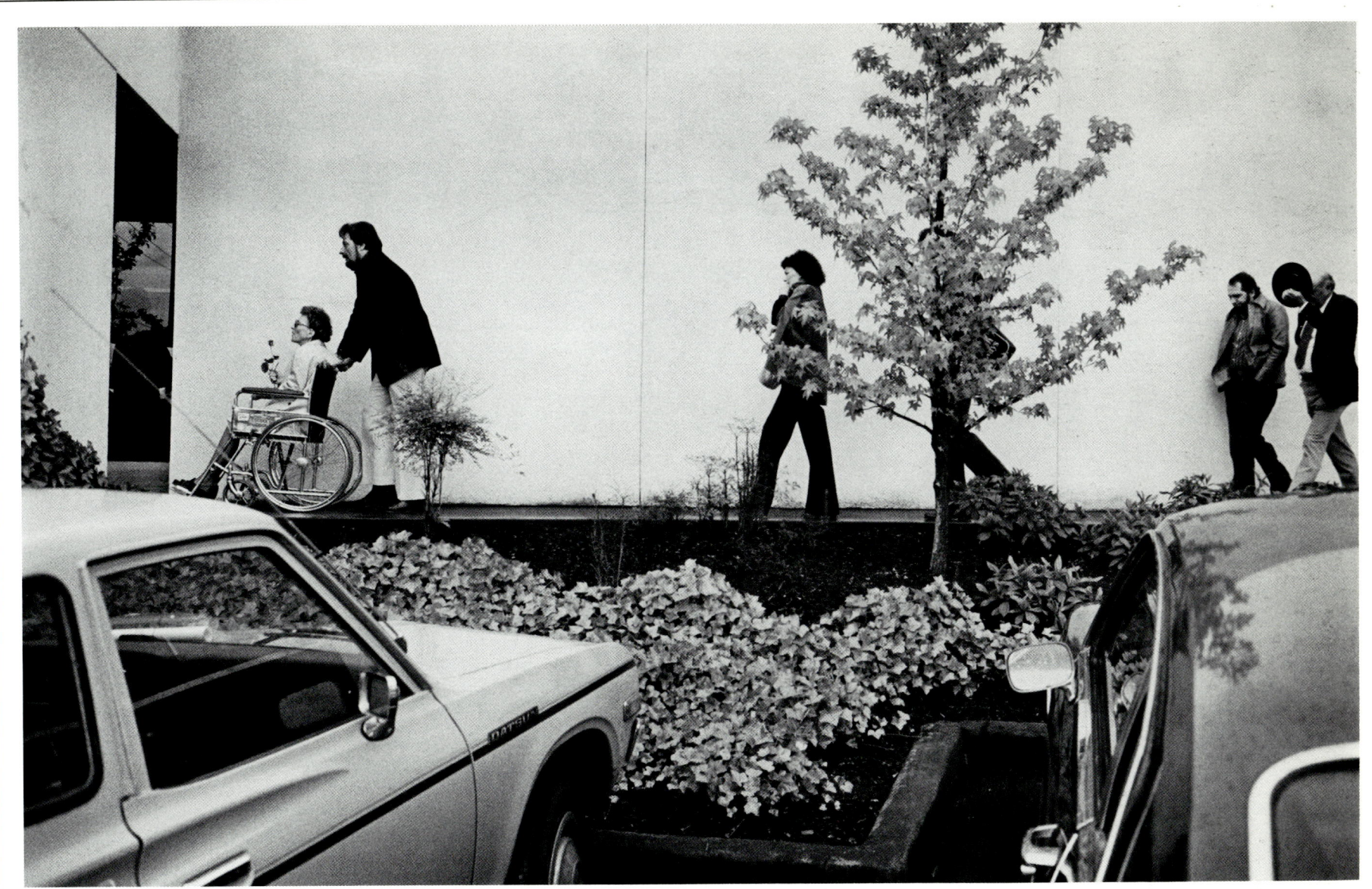

After a year at the nursing home, Genevieve passed away. Donnabelle took responsibility for the funeral plans and notified relatives and friends. Donnabelle arranged to have the local preacher deliver the eulogy. He visited Donnabelle the night before the funeral to familiarize himself with Genevieve's life. The funeral provided an opportunity for the first family reunion in years.

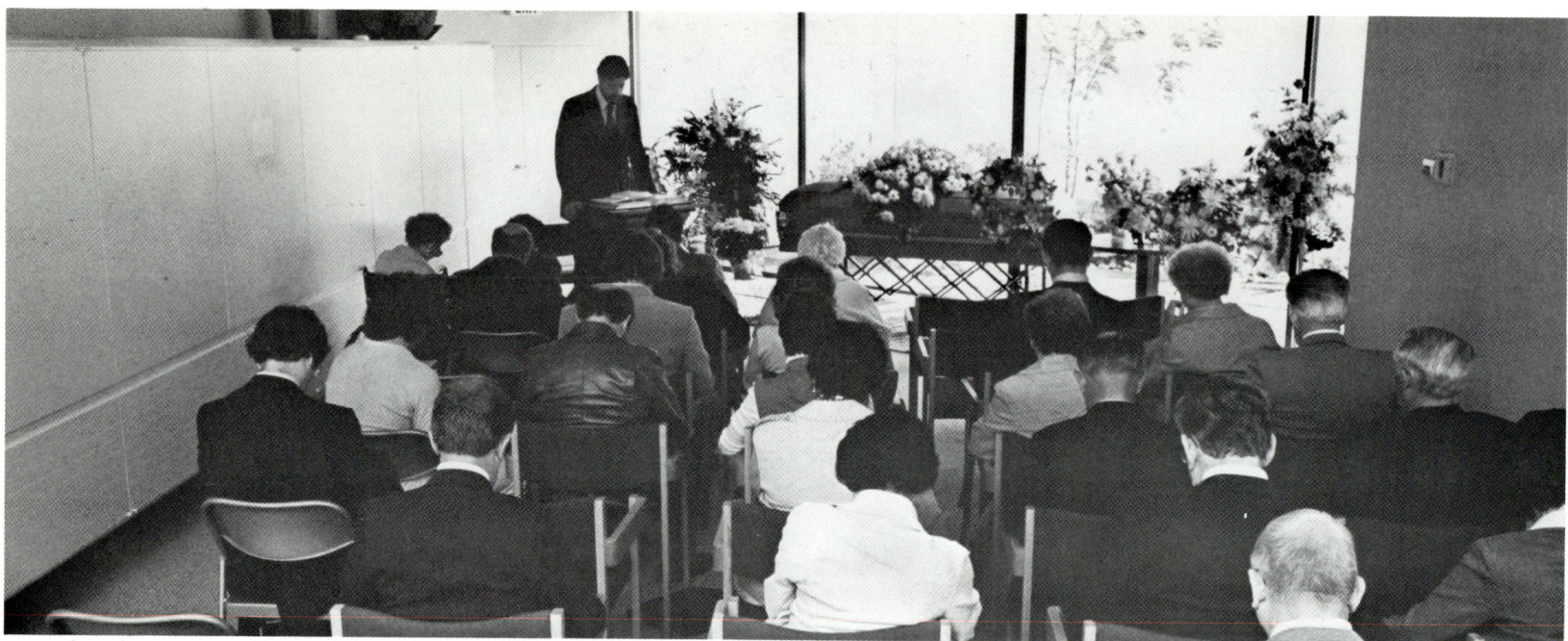

Genevieve was 81 years old when she died. She is survived by her child, Donnabelle, who I had the opportunity to be with last night.

A person's life, 81 years, should make a great impact on people. I know that Genevieve did have that kind of impact. She wasn't a complex person in the sense that you would think, but one with simple tastes, a simple nature. Donnabelle commented last night that there were two things Genevieve liked to do very much. She liked to bake, she liked to cook, and she liked to bake for her husband. She was busy doing the things that her husband liked the most. The other thing that she liked to do was that she liked to crochet. I don't think there was a day that went by when Donnabelle was a young child that she didn't have some beautiful crochet for her. She was devoted to her husband. Devoted to her children. Devoted to making the life in her home the best it could possibly be.

Last night, after I left Donnabelle, I went home and thought about what she had told me about her mother. One of the things I would like to speculate about is what would Genevieve say to us, if by some miracle she could come back this morning and speak to us. What would she really hold important? What would she communicate about what she learned in death? What would it be?

I came up with two things. Number one, she would say take the time to stop and smell the roses. We live in a high-pressured world, where it seems like our personal lives are squeezed into a few precious seconds. Often our awareness becomes dim and stilted. When you lose sight of beauty, you lose sight of people, and you lose the sight of those special moments.

I think the second thing Genevieve would tell us is that God gave us a family for a purpose. He put us with this group of people for a reason. The reason is that He figures that they are the best group of people to help us grow, mature and develop. . . . He gave us a family to help us remember, to give us a sense of continuity, to be able to look back on the past, and to see where we came from and where we are going.

Today our society does us and our families a disfavor. Our families are splintered and scattered, driven apart, because we don't take the time to touch base with those who are the most important and closest to us. Sometimes misunderstandings occur, causing bitterness and resentment. These misunderstandings may become locked up. I think if Genevieve were sitting here today, she would say: "If you've got something that is wrong between you and your family, get it out, say it, before it's too late."

—Reverend Richard

GEORGIA

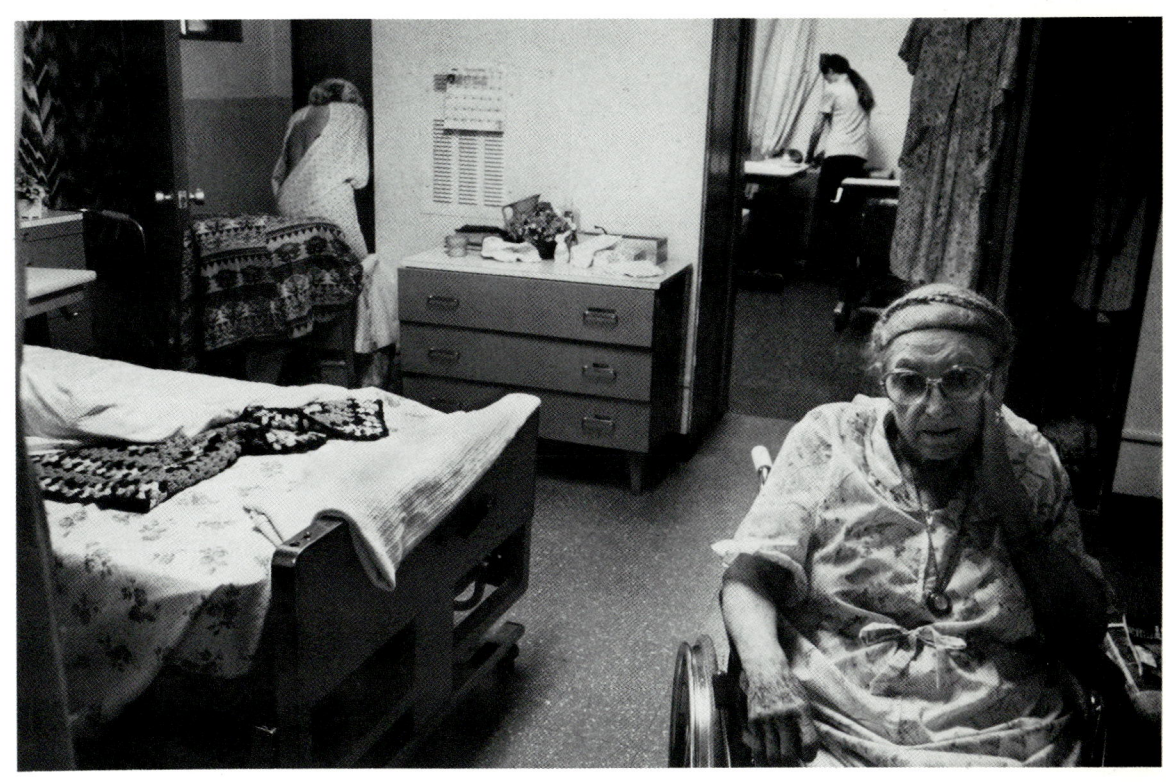

Georgia entered the nursing home following hospitalization for surgery. Upon arrival, she immediately had trouble with her assigned roommate. She complained to the Administrator, and was moved to another room.

Georgia has always known how to handle herself. In the thirties, she worked in a number of beer saloons, and was adept in dealing with unruly customers. "They'd walk in, with their heads up in the air like they were the only stud in the country. I never rang up the register when they ordered. I'd give 'em their beer and if they started getting smart I would grab their beer off the counter and pour it down the drain. I'd slap their money back on the counter and say, 'There's the door.'"

I'd been in the hospital many times, but they never said anything about goin' to a nursing home. That's what happened to me and I never thought it would happen.

I had gangrene in my legs, and where you got gangrene you just rot. My sister signed the legal release so the doctor could take them off. At first I couldn't adjust to it, but you don't die when you want to. If you did, there'd be a hell of a lot of dead people. So you just go on fighting this war.

I was thinking of getting my own place and paying somebody to take care of me. I'm not that hard to take care of. But you just can't trust people anymore. They might take off and leave you by yourself. I know of old people who have been dead for three or four days before anybody found 'em. I had a friend who lived by herself, and one day she fell down and couldn't get to the phone. She lay on the floor for three days before anybody heard her hollering.

My sister asked me to live with her, but I wouldn't. I didn't want to be a burden to her. Why should she take an old woman like me with no legs? She has a right to live her life as she wants. But I'm not going to give up as long as there is any breath in my body. I'm going to fight. You only go down this road once, and I'm not going to come back and go down it again. I will adjust to whatever the situation is around here.

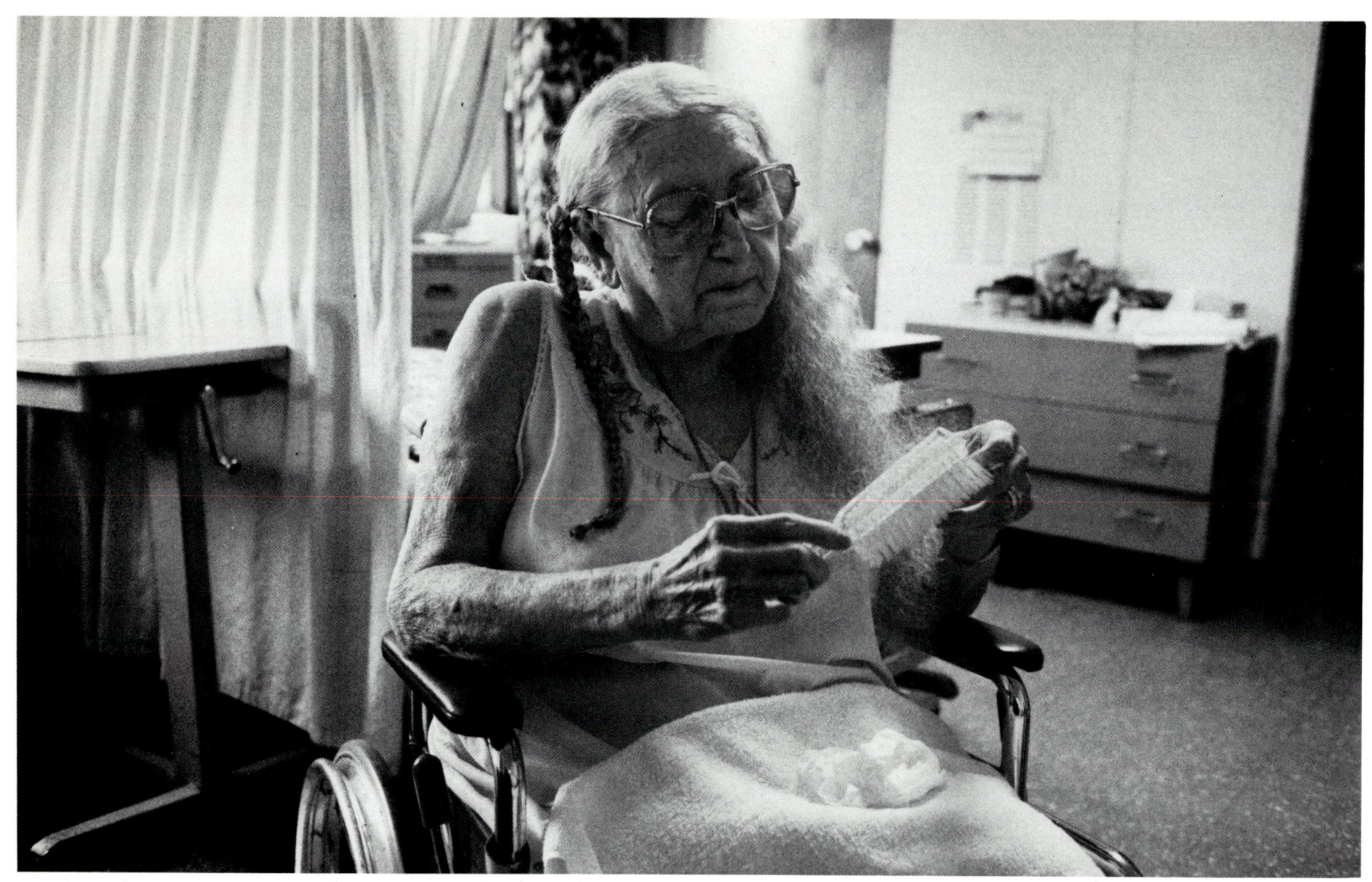

I don't use the nightgowns they give you around here. I've got my own. The ones they give you are open at the back, so when you go to the bathroom everybody can see your behind from here to Timbuctu. They look vulgar too. They don't do anything for a woman's shape. Not that I have anything to show—but who wants to go around in those things? As long as I've got my own, I'm gonna wear them.

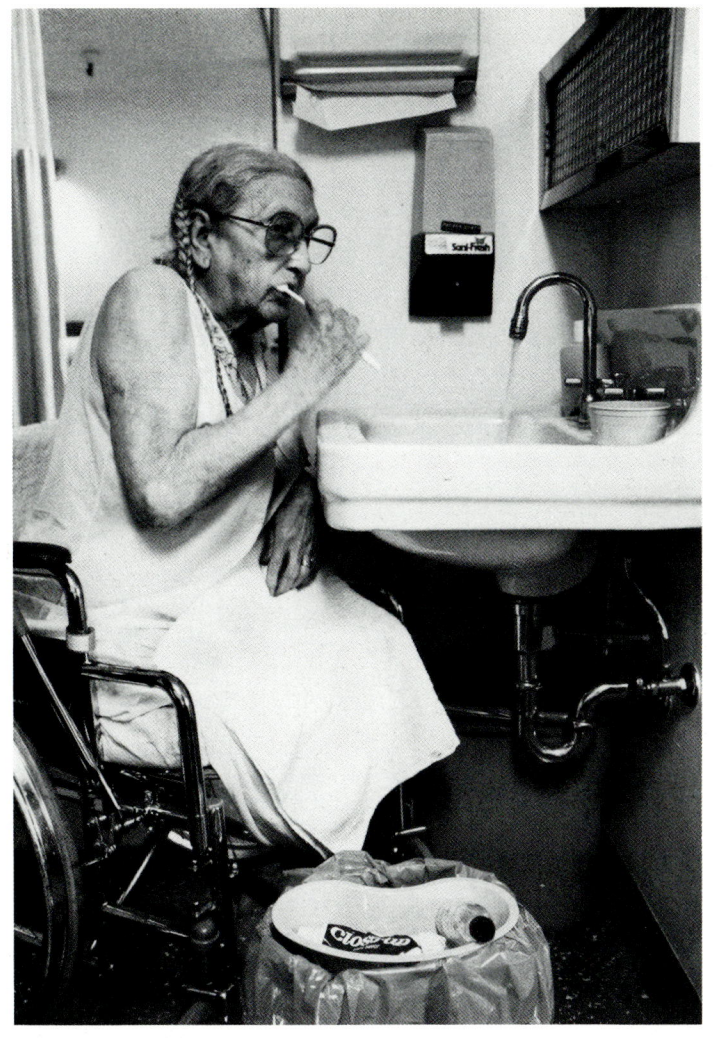 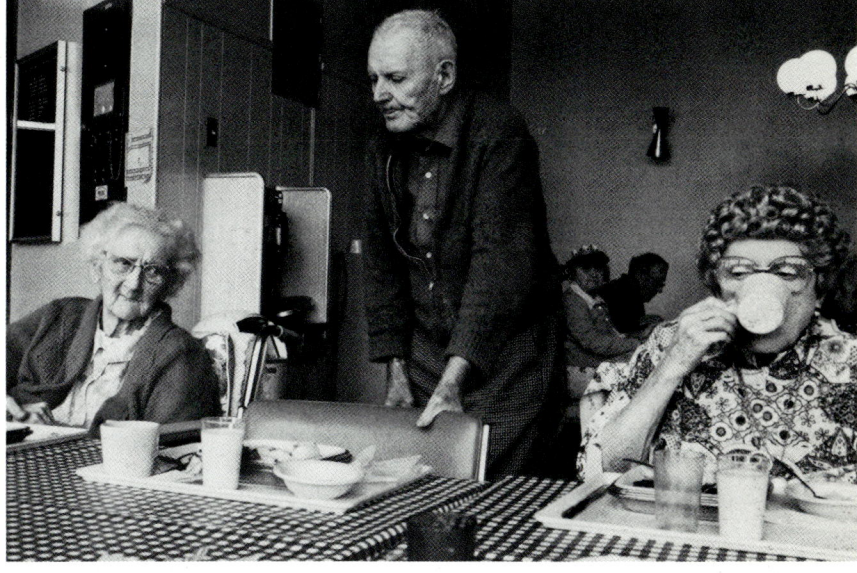

Every morning I have to go to the next room to use the washbasin. There are two ladies in there as well as three in this room. Five people for one washbasin. My roommate takes a sponge bath every morning, standing there naked and bathing herself. There just isn't any privacy. You can't say, "Get out of here, I want to use the washbasin." I don't use it any more than I have to. That way I can keep the peace with the rest of them.

If that man had been in his office last night, I don't know what his name is—you know, the guy who runs this place—I would've took the tray they set in front of me, set it down in his office and said, "O.K., you son-of-a-bitch, you eat it!"

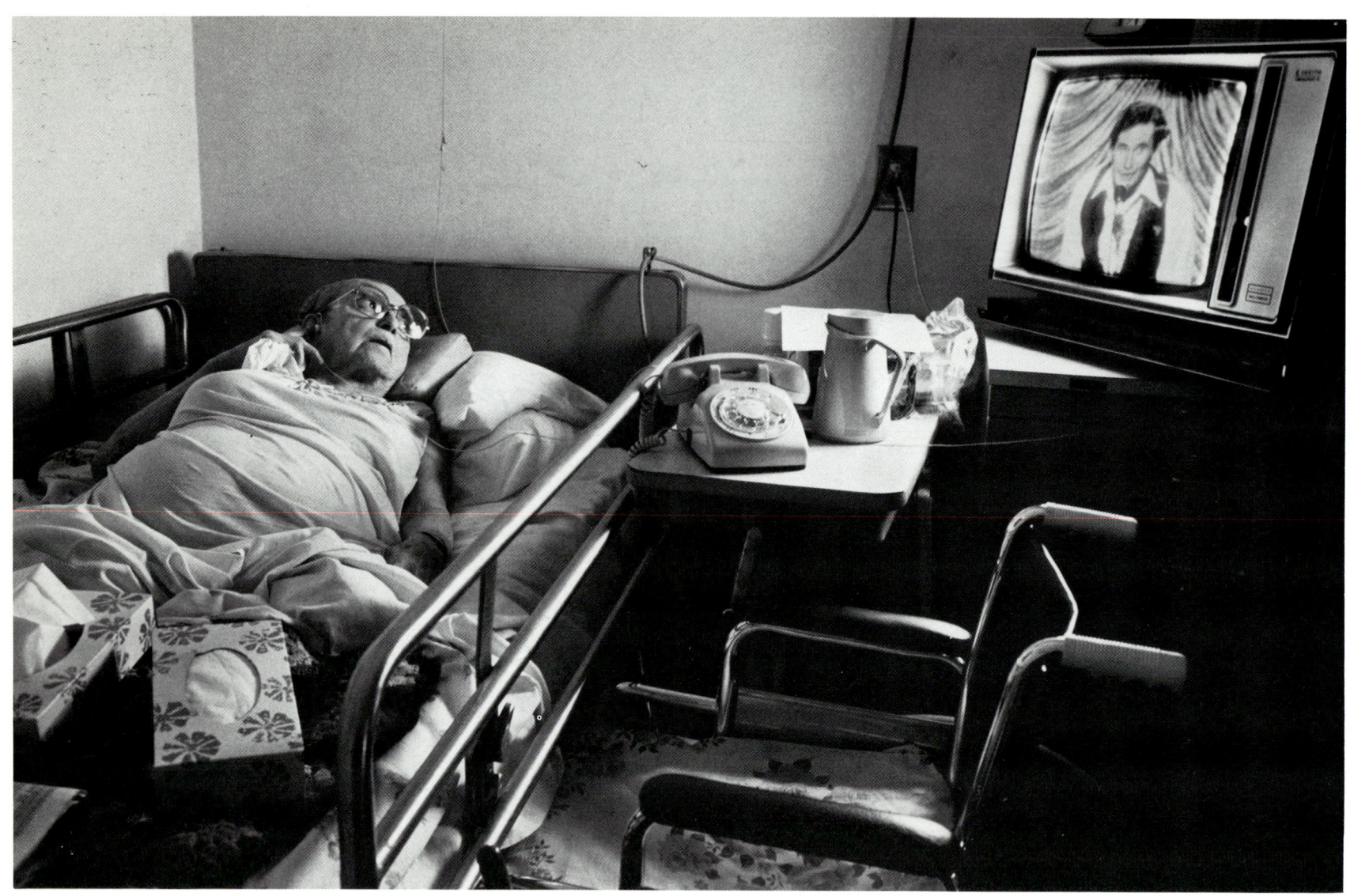

The first couple of weeks around here were very lonely. I had to get on by myself. Nobody came and talked to me. It was sink or swim. So I spent my time reading the paper and watching TV. What the hell else do you do when you don't know anybody?

—Georgia

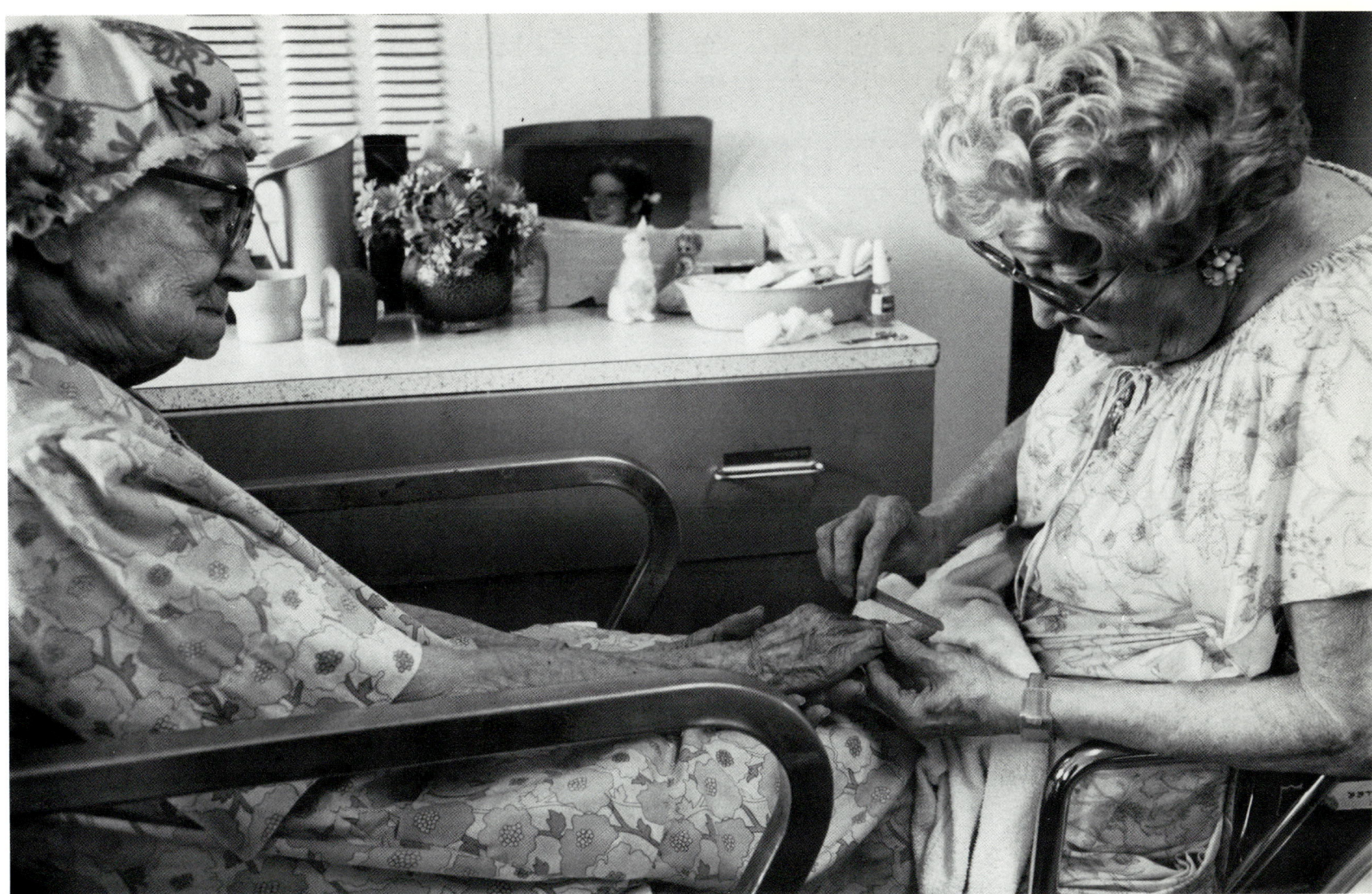

Mattie reminds me of my mother. I took care of Mother for eight years before she died, and she got to be a skinny little old lady like Mattie. She was a fussy woman too, just like Mattie. The way you hear poor Mattie gripe sometimes, you'd think that she lived at the Hilton. She wants everything so damn perfect. She's awfully particular about her nails, but I enjoy doing them for her.

When anybody around here bothers Mattie, it makes me awfully mad. The old biddy next door raises a stink every time Mattie uses the washbasin, and the other day she threatened to hit her. If that old biddy does anything to Mattie, I'll knock her down. I started out with a devil when I first moved into this place, but I wound up with an angel.

—Georgia

FRANK AND ROSA

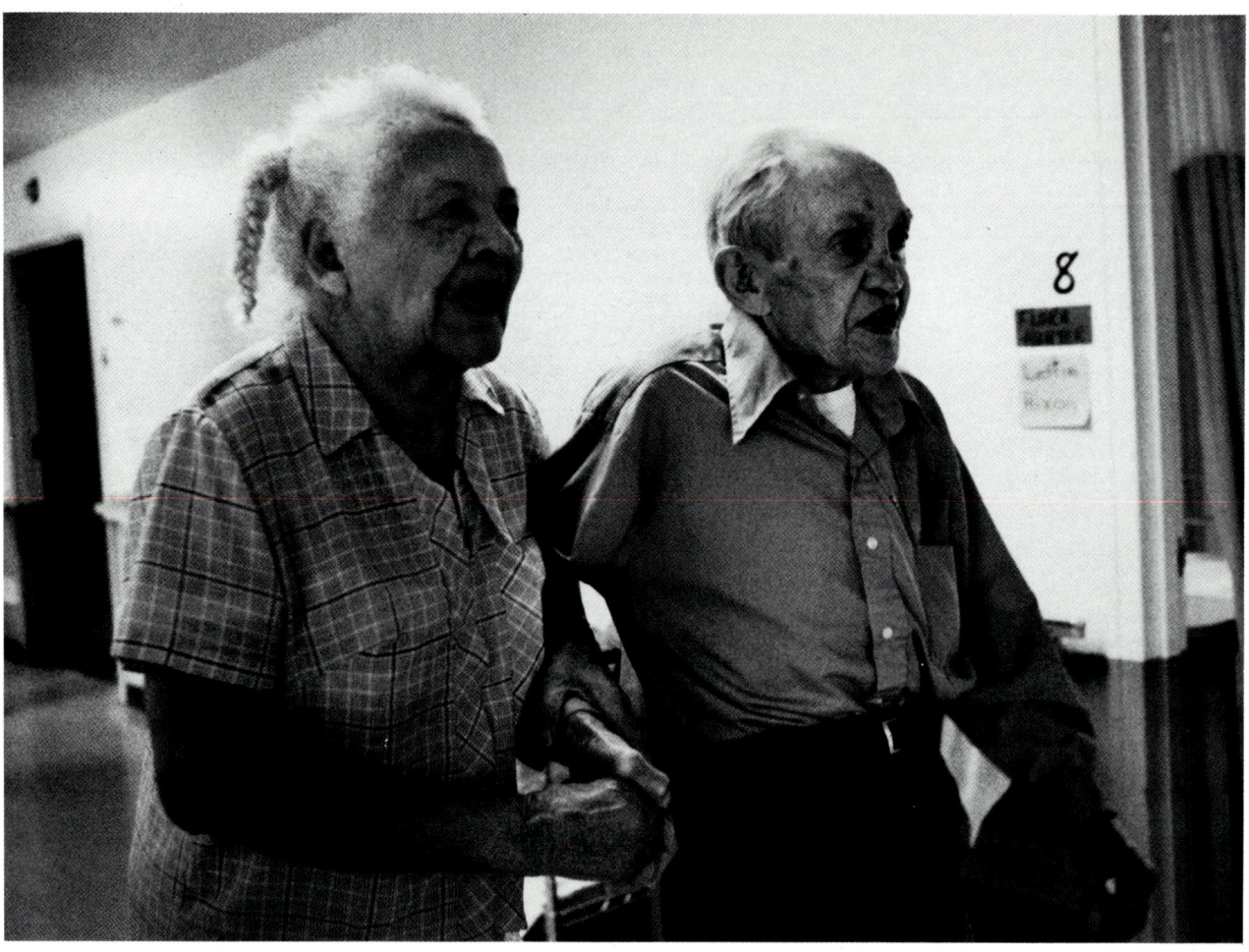

For most of his life, Frank had been a skid row alcoholic. When he first came to the nursing home, he largely kept to himself. According to his younger sister's friend, who had known Frank for most of his life, "He was a foul-mouthed, mean-spirited drunk who was nothin' but trouble." But there was a different side to Frank. In the nursing home, he developed a strong relationship for the first time in his life. Over several months, Rosa, who is blind, and Frank became very close. Frank's health improved to the point where he no longer needed nursing care and, according to the guidelines set by the Welfare Department, he had to leave.

I've known Frank for quite a while. They put me over beside him in the dining room, and he helped me to eat. He would butter my bread and fix my food. He was very nice to me. I couldn't see my way back to my room and I asked Frank if he had eyes to take me. At first he didn't think he could. I asked him why not. And so it got so he took me all the time. And he didn't let anyone else take me. I felt happy that someone thought enough of me to take me along. During the summertime, he would take me outside for a walk. And he would talk to me all the time. He said that he loved me. I really miss Frank now that he is gone. I think of him every day, wondering what he is doing.

—Rosa

When Frank's health improved, he was transferred from the nursing home to a hotel for the aged that offered a lesser level of care. Frank didn't like the place. It was a catch-as-catch-can geriatric welfare hotel—the residents, discarded pensioners biding their time. Every time we visited, his mood had become more sullen and bitter. He rarely talked about Rosa and when we brought a message from her, he would pretend he didn't care. Shortly after our last visit, he started drinking again.

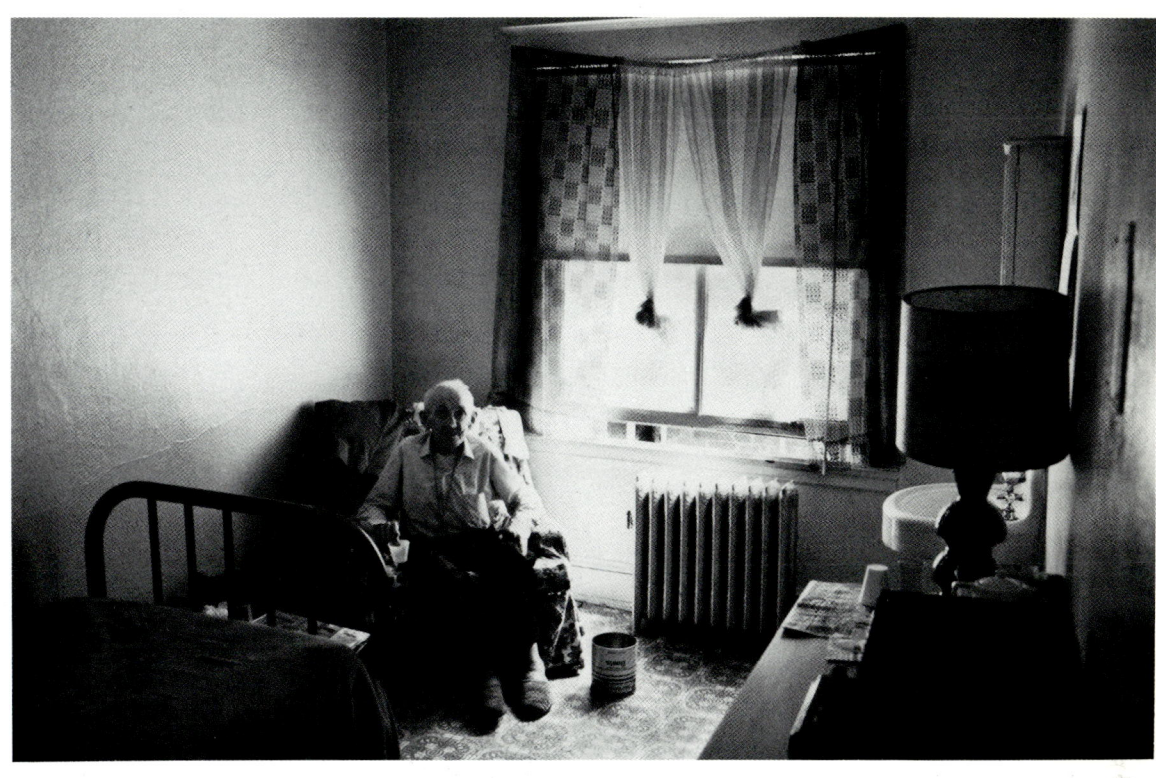

I'm telling you, they don't do a darn thing for you around here. They don't ask how you are doing. Over at the nursing home they looked after you. They bathed my feet with salt water and did other things that you needed. Here you could be dead for four days and they would say, "Gee, what stinks around here?"

My room has got a pound of cockroaches. They're in every room—every room. I told the woman who cleans to get rid of 'em. "They're hard to get rid of," she said. "You better get rid of them," I told her, "or otherwise I'm going to get the health people to look into the matter." The bugs are driving me crazy. They start a runnin' around the room like it's a racetrack. I don't like stepping on the son-of-a-guns. They're hard and so damn fat. I'll swat 'em with a paper and then I'll put them into the sink, and give them a doggone good cold bath—the last they'll ever get. Or sometimes I'll boil up some water and give 'em a hot bath.

They're gyppin' me here, stealing my allowance. When I sign my welfare checks for $200 or sometimes even $300, I says, "Now where's my allowance?" And she says, "Only a dollar a day." I'd like to chop that owner's hand off! Mash her in the mouth. I know what I'd get—I'd get the penitentiary. But I'd be better off there than this damn dump. She's lower than a snake belly in a ten-foot well. She's nothin' but a black snake. The devil herself, that's what she is.

Hotels, hospitals, nursing homes—how many nursing homes do you think I've been in? I've been in about six of them. Yeah, six nursing homes. Jesus Christ, I was in this bed, I was in that bed. From one to the other, I made my rounds. Half the time I didn't know who I was anymore. I just made my rounds—I'd be here, there, it was a merry-go-round. I'm telling you I wouldn't go through all that again if you gave me half the money in the world.

—Frank

MINNIE

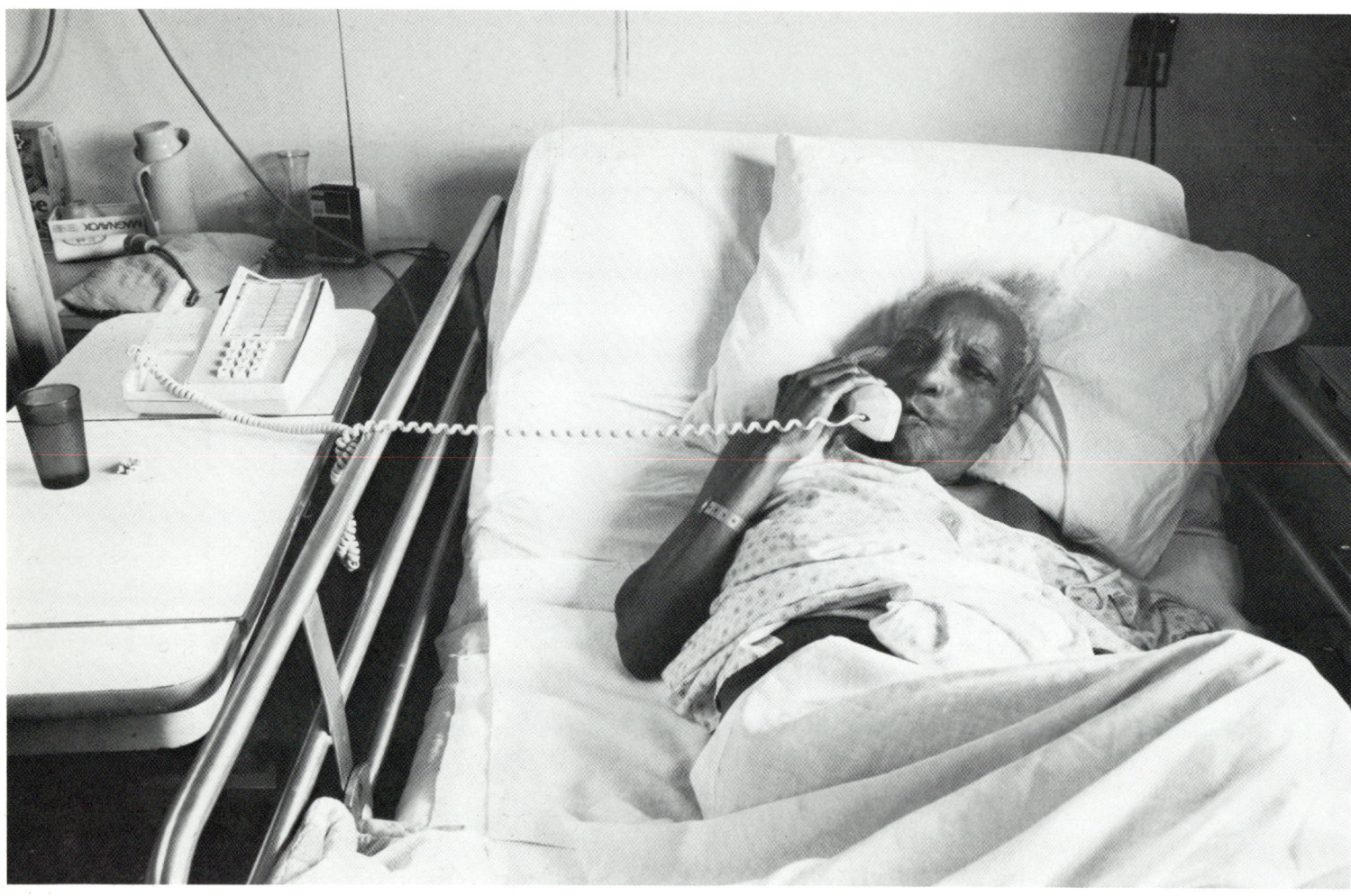

One day Rob and I heard the distinctive voice of William F. Buckley coming from one of the rooms on South hall. Curious, we went inside. "Boys, that guy Buckley must be pretty smart if all he does is talk to people on TV," said a peppery black woman, pointing toward her Sony television.

Before her stroke, Minnie was an active woman and had many contacts in the community. She worked as a cook for a prominent family for twenty-five years and in her spare time was active in her social service club, The Modern Matrons. Minnie stays in touch with her family and her many friends by telephone. Her phone is programmed with eighteen phone numbers, so all she has to do is touch a button. Often she will spend over two hours a day on the phone. "I'd be sunk without that phone," says Minnie.

It's terrible to be in a situation like this—not being able to do what you're used to doing all of your life. If this place caught fire I couldn't get out of here unless somebody helped me. That's a bad feeling. That's a feeling that'll make you have nightmares. Even though I'm in this shape, I'm grateful 'cause God has been good to me. I'm lucky. Most old people are just thrown out. People just ignore old folks, stick 'em in places like this and never come to see 'em. I see this with my own eyes. People still love to come and talk to me. I have visitors 'til I'm tired of them—except for my family. My family is the most important thing to me. Everybody says, boy, you've got it made. My family comes to see me, they bring me food, they bring me clothes, they bring me presents. Some people have wall-to-wall carpet. Me, I got wall-to-wall love.

—Minnie

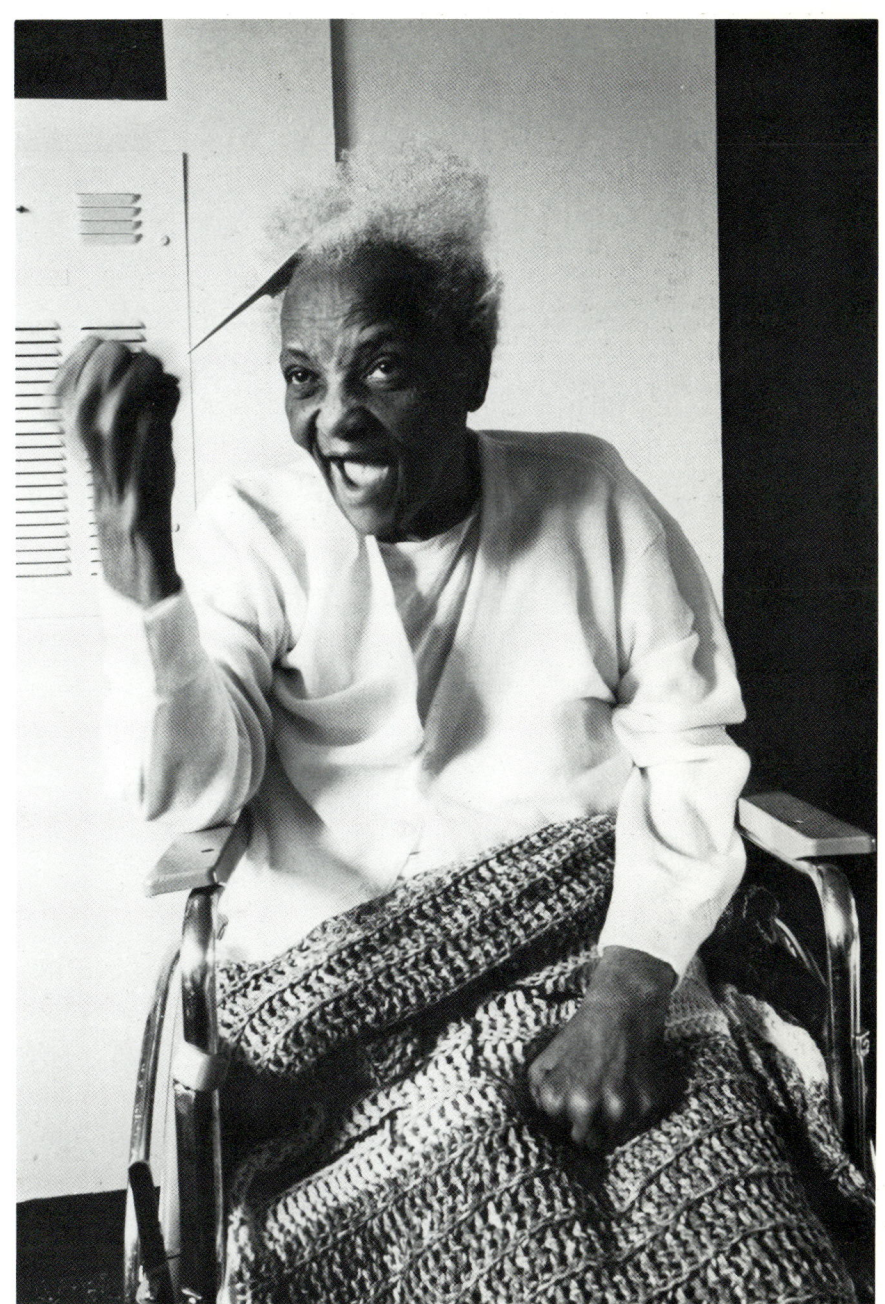

III. Caretakers

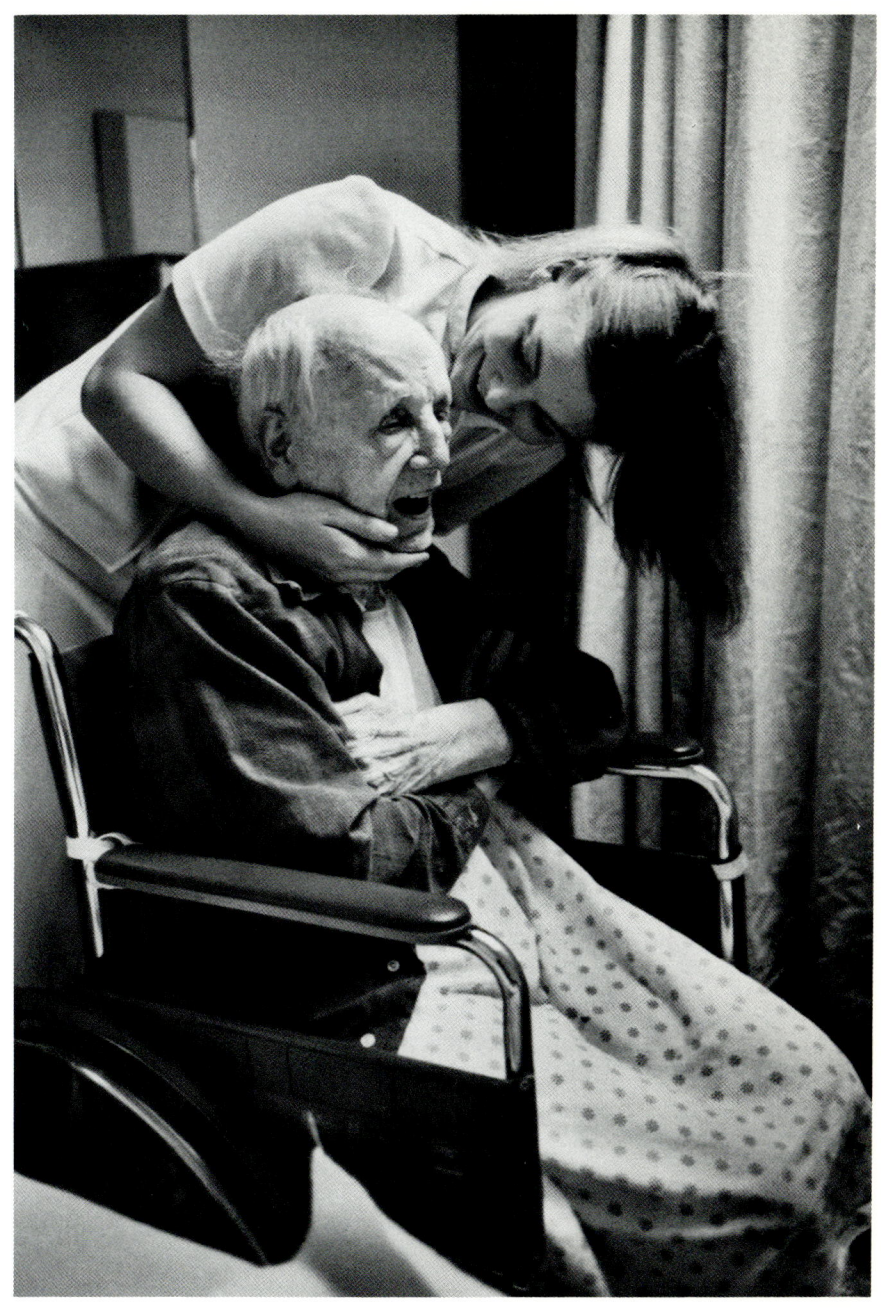

SHIRLEY

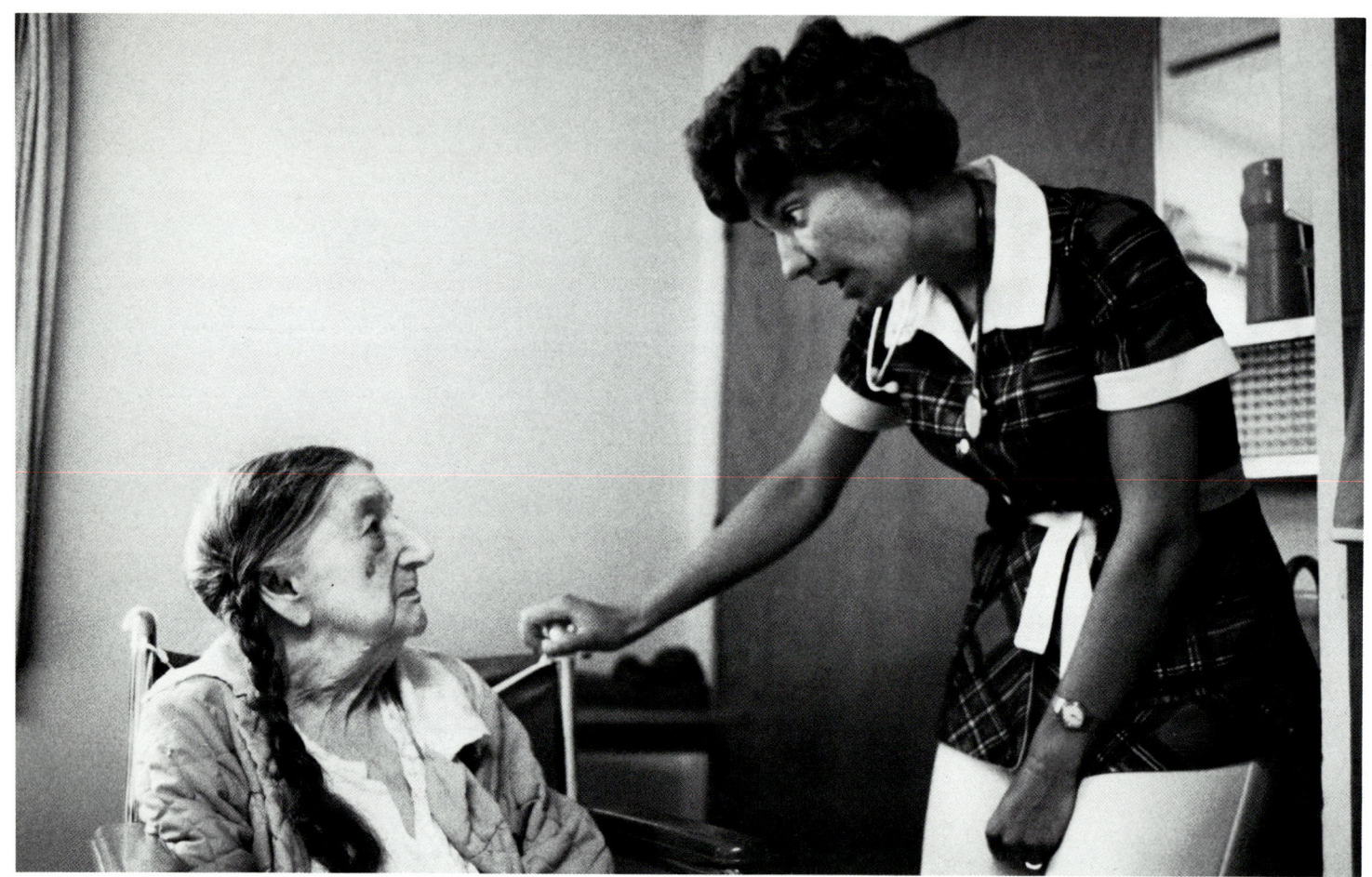

Shirley, a former nun, has been the home's Director of Nursing for over three years. Away from the nursing home, she seems like an ordinary person; in the nursing home, Shirley represents a kind of sanctuary from the often rough-and-tumble existence. A steady procession of residents seek her out during the course of her twelve-hour day. She will stop whatever she is doing to come close and gaze intently into a person's eyes. When a resident unload's her troubles, Shirley seems to listen with all of her senses, and knows what to say. The residents love her. And she loves them.

I've always been interested in missions, and I feel I am in a missionary field. Nursing is very very fulfilling; I've never regretted it. I've been to nursing homes that are pretty well-to-do and have everything, but I feel that my mission is in the welfare homes. That's where the real need is.

When I first arrived here, the home was all mixed up. I saw immediately that one of the things that had to happen was that there had to be some structure, some organization. Within a month we had a mass moving day, where almost everybody changed rooms. I felt we had prepared the residents—I felt we really did—but the first night a lady died for no known reason, and the Doctor and I felt it was attributable to transfer trauma. The woman who passed away was the kind of person who didn't speak her mind, and who had no one to intercede for her. So I learned the hard way that you really think before you move a person, and you really do a lot of preparation with them.

Each day I ask myself, "Are we still striving towards our goals of giving optimum care with what we have and providing a good home for our residents?" Working in my position is like putting out fires all the time. If you don't like to put out fires, you shouldn't be doing this. Throughout the day I try to recognize if things are wrong. I'm not a person who's great at telling people, "My, you've done a good job today. I appreciate you so much." I don't like that kind of false praise. But I do think it's important to help out if you have any extra time, to show the staff I'm willing to pitch in.

Probably the biggest frustration for the residents is the lack of privacy. I would find it very very difficult to live in the space they have to live in. There's nowhere in the building where they can shut the door and be by themselves. Nowhere. Many of the residents come from the hospital where they have been treated for hypertension, and here they are put in a situation which causes more hypertension. It doesn't make sense.

Some of the residents don't get visitors except on the first of the month, when their Social Security check comes. That's twenty-five dollars for personal expenses that they're not able to spend. So families can come in and take the money. At least it brings them in. One woman's daughter dropped her off the day after Christmas and has never been back. I just can't understand a person doing that. I get angry. But I suppose that if they're that type of person, it's probably better that we're taking care of their parents.

—Shirley

KEN

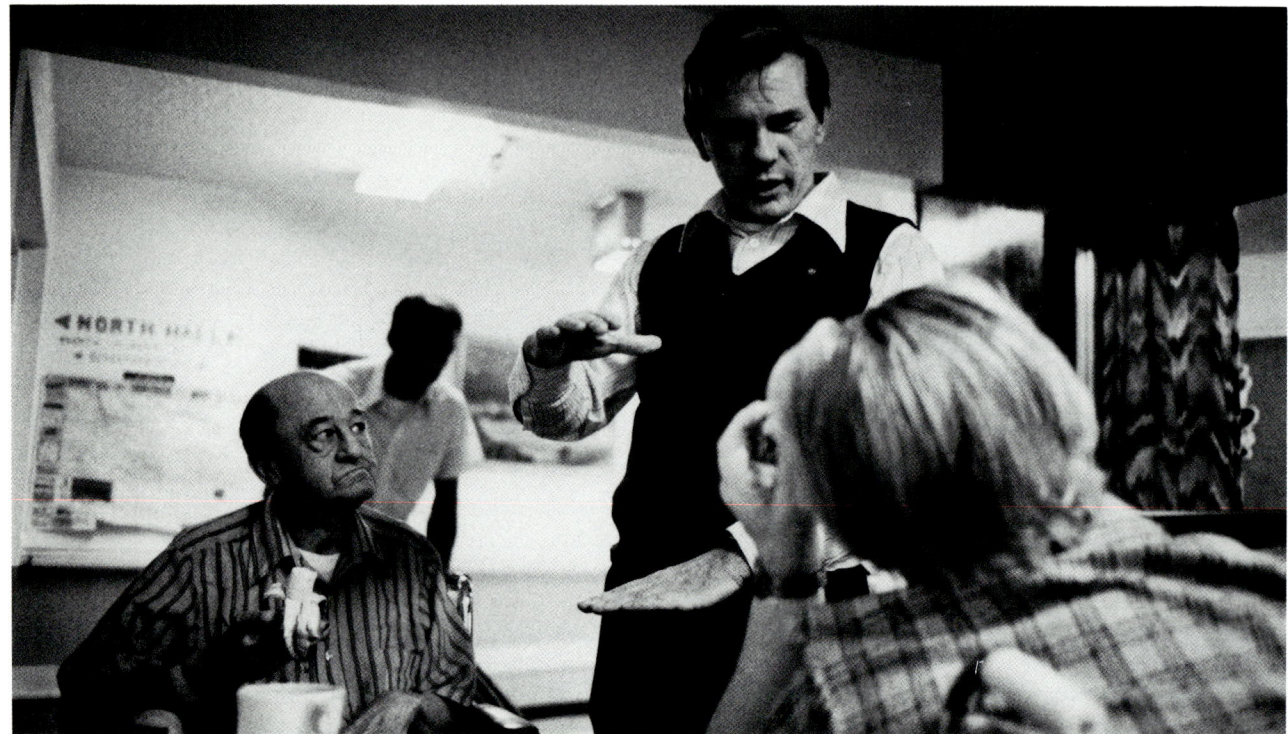

As a nursing home administrator, Ken daily faces irreconcilable problems: chronic understaffing, profit-making pressures, family complaints, and contradictory rules and regulations. His ability and concern show clearly as he works to minimize conflicts and create the best home possible for the residents. In spite of the pressures, his sense of humor often surfaces—a welcome relief from the sobering realities of the nursing home.

Unlike many of his colleagues, Ken maintains an open door policy. The media and visitors are encouraged to visit the nursing home—even when it may not be in his best interest. On one media visit, Ken looked pained as he watched a local television crew traverse North and East halls, ignoring the residents who were positioned in their doorways ogling the "TV people." Rubbing his forehead, Ken murmured, "You know, any number of things can go wrong, and if we get some bad publicity, it could wreck the hell out of our census."

I have been a nursing home administrator for seven years. I first got interested in nursing homes when I worked at the VA Hospital as a staff nurse. Many of our patients who came in were from nursing homes, and they had a lot of problems. I wondered what the devil was going on in those places. As an administrator, now I know. It's one crisis after another, and there's no end to it. You get your nurse aides up to staffing level, you get your RNs up to staffing level—you got everything stabilized—and then you lose a cook. Or you lose a housekeeper. Then you got problems in the laundry 'cause nobody wants to take shit out of diapers and pads and soak them for minimum wage. Before you know it, the whole damn cycle starts over again.

When it comes to staffing, economics is the name of the game. I can't demand the kind of aides I need 'cause I can't afford to pay them the wages they're worth. I can't compete with the hospitals. I can't even afford to pay my licensed nurses fifteen thousand a year—what the city pays someone to pick leaves out of the park.

We have a very unfair system. The state will give you money for a hearing evaluation, but no money for a hearing aid; or they will give you money for a dental examination, but no money for the dental work. Why even have the evaluation if you can't do anything about it? Why even waste the money? What's really sad is if you go on welfare, the state is going to strip you of everything you have. You lose your self-respect, your dignity, and your ability to function as a human being. You get $25 a month for personal funds irrespective of your personal needs. If you need a hearing aid or eyeglasses, you're out of luck, unless you have a family concerned enough to pay your way. If you smoke—for crying out loud—with the way cigarettes cost, and if you smoke a carton a week, there's no way you are going to be able to survive. Because by the time you've smoked, gotten a haircut for four or five dollars—assuming you don't want an aide to cut your hair—you're broke. You don't even have enough money to go out and buy yourself a hamburger. . . .

When it comes to the old, society just doesn't give a damn. The attitude is: the hell with these people, they have lived their lives, so why put any more money into them. They're 86 years old, let them die. But the numbers of aged are increasing by leaps and bounds. The younger people are producing fewer children, and the working people have less capital to subsidize the older folks. Take the old man of a number of years ago. He had a retirement pension and savings, which combined were enough for nursing home costs. But for most of us that is no longer adequate. It has to do with inflation. The retirement programs are just not able to support people. More and more middle class people are goin' welfare.

In my own small way, I'm trying to turn this around. I realize that someday maybe I will be in a nursing home, and I hope to God that what changes I can make in this crazy system will make it a better place tomorrow. But when I get families calling me up saying, "Gee, Ken, what a great job you're doing for my mother," this gives me a warm feeling inside. To me this is what makes it all worthwhile.

—Ken

RICHARD

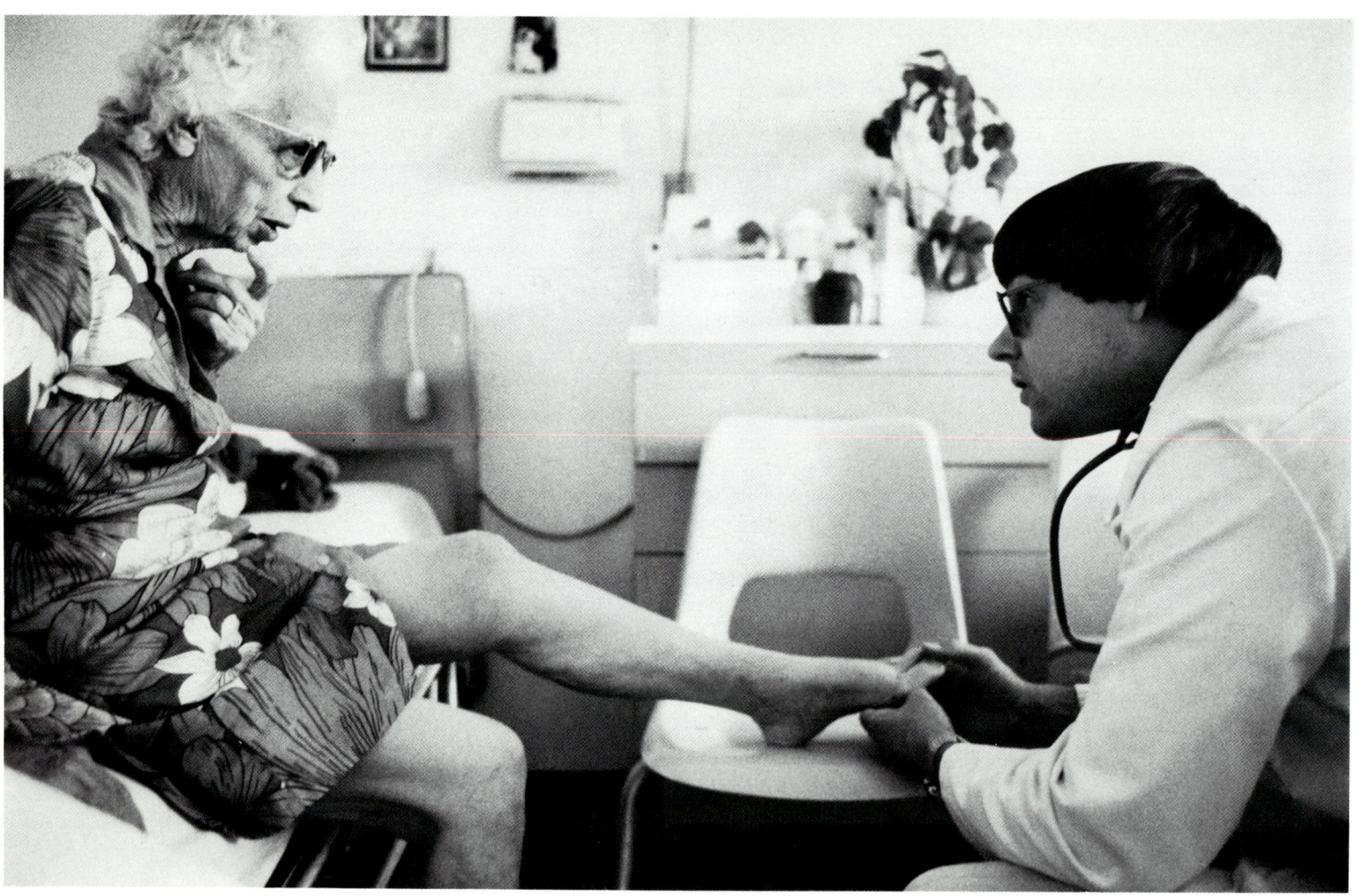

Richard was the house physician when we first came to the nursing home. He believes that understanding and compassion are indispensable allies to medical treatment, and his patients responded well to his care. When he had to leave the nursing home unexpectedly, many of his patients, in a rare display of unity, wrote letters and signed a petition asking for his return.

When I first started at the nursing home, I found it a strange, chaotic environment. It was frightening, and I didn't know what was causing the fear and the strangeness. In retrospect, however, I now understand some of those very intense feelings. On my first day, I was given responsibility for sixty-three patients. As a doctor I felt threatened because I realized that I wasn't going to be able to cure all those people. With all the skills of my profession, I could not heal them and save them from dying. In a nursing home you are bombarded by that reality every day.

This nursing home provides a good environment, largely because they don't rely too heavily on drugs. The use of tranquilizers in many cases is appropriate, but only at the proper dosage. The dosage should allow the patient to remain active and do as many things for himself as he can. If the patients sometimes get upset or anxious, well, that's fine, because you and I sometimes get upset or anxious. A resident may yell or fume or sulk or swear, and it's not considered inappropriate. I do not get excessive requests to sedate patients here.

I like the concept of being specialized and a rarity in my profession. There are very few good geriatricians; I will be a good one someday. I am now learning those skills. But first the concept of being a geriatrician must be upgraded. Right now there's a stigma attached to working in nursing home situations. Initially I felt like I should apologize for what I was doing. It took me a long time to develop pride in this work.

From my background as a family doctor, I know that taking care of nursing home residents means more than just diagnosing heart disease or Parkinson's disease. It means somehow assimilating all that these people are going through and trying somehow to uplift them. I do a lot of touching with my patients—holding their hand or putting my hand on their shoulder. That's important to both of us. Somehow there is that need. There are things I've learned from practicing at the nursing home that help me in practicing medicine in other environments, and that have helped me in becoming a better human being. I've learned how to interact with someone who has trouble communicating rationally, or how to interact with someone who is overwhelmed by the misery of their situation. You realize that as a doctor you don't belong on a pedestal; you simply have been given the privilege of being a very special part of another person's life.

—Richard

LONNIE

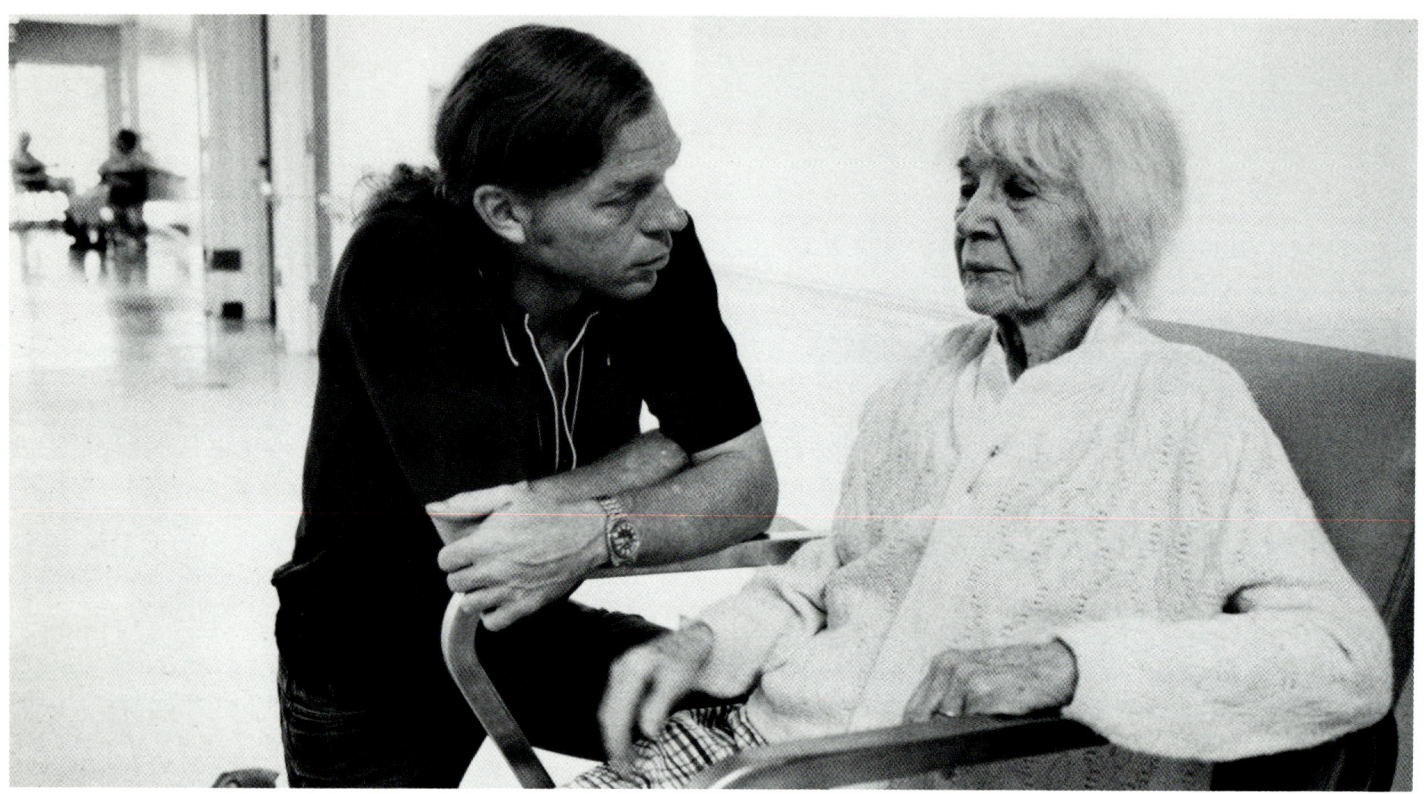

Officially employed by the Oregon Welfare Department as a caseworker for Medicaid patients, Lonnie is also politically active in nursing home reform. He attends many of the legislative committees on aging and is often called to testify. Recently he was offered an administrative position by the state, but he turned it down. He didn't want to lose contact with the residents.

Skeptical of our presence at the nursing home, Lonnie kept a vigilant eye on us for the first three months. When it became evident that we weren't muckrakers, he became a strong advocate for our work and a close friend.

Never one to get ruffled, Lonnie is a steadying influence at the nursing home, especially during a crisis. Fiercely protective of his clients, he will, when necessary, fight with the state to obtain the best possible advantage for the residents and their families.

When I first started working for Welfare, the only position open was in a nursing home. At the time, working in a nursing home as a caseworker was pretty much like being shipped to Siberia. It really didn't matter if you were incompetent. Residents were "losers" and there wasn't much significant work that could be done in a nursing home. All that was required was to keep the paper work flowing. . . .

I found nursing homes pretty frightening at first. It was the deadness of those places that really bothered me. Whatever hopes the patients might once have had were gone. They were no longer human beings, but objects waiting to die. I felt that my own energy was sapped by these patients. I would do what I had to do in there as quickly as possible and get the hell out. I told my supervisor that as soon as a transfer became available I was going to hike.

Clearly I forgot to hike.

I decided I wasn't going to content myself just drifting in, looking at the charts and getting out. I began to spend time in the facility getting to know the residents and staff. What I discovered was that there is a great similarity between the people here and the outside world. That the one hundred and twenty residents here are not just a figure but represent a hundred and twenty different sets of values, of ideas, of ways of dealing with reality. . . .

Although I find the bureaucratic aspect of working in a nursing home somewhat absurd, I try to float with the rules and regulations. I have studied the manuals and know them thoroughly. Now many caseworkers say the manuals are bullshit, that they're continually changing and there's no point in learning them. But the better I know them the more benefit I can be to my clients.

I feel that I have an obligation to do as many good things for the residents as I can, so I have willingly stuck myself into this system. Maybe I have delusions of grandeur, that I can come in here and make a difference. But all you ever get are the little victories, like working out a roommate problem. The things that residents constantly complain about—the food, the lack of privacy, the lack of space—I can't change. It's easy for me to get frustrated, and even angry, with clients who continually complain about these things, but they only want conditions that anyone should have.

I guess then that I'm as caught up in the system as anyone else. I'm a victim, but a willing victim, just as are all the nurses, aides, administrators, and anyone else who works in a long-term care situation. The difference is that we can opt out; the residents can't.

—Lonnie

CAROL

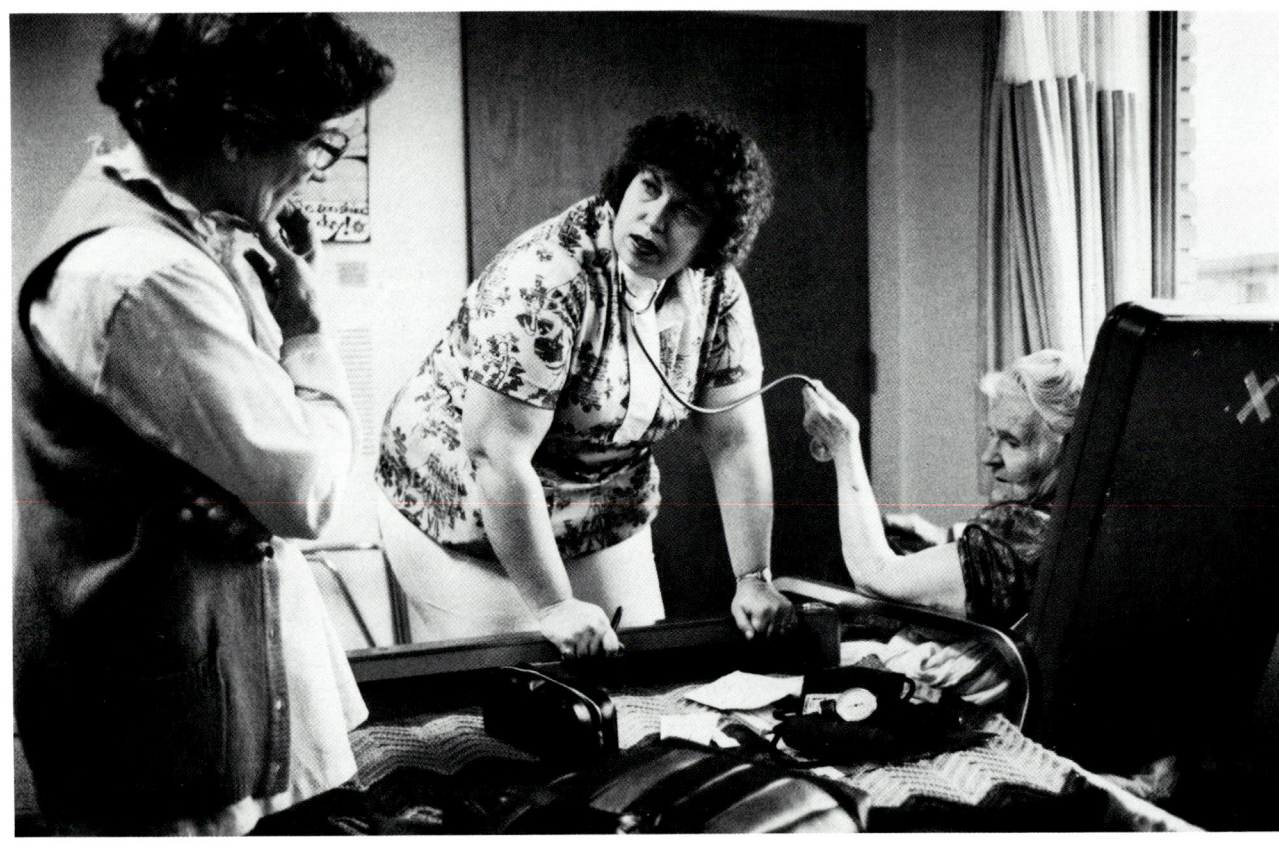

Carol is like a veteran cop on a beat. She has an intimate knowledge of all the idiosyncracies of the residents on her section as well as an instinctive feel for the day-to-day rhythms of the nursing home. When things become frenzied, which is especially difficult when there's only a skeleton crew, Carol is unflappable as she rallies the younger, less experienced aides in completing work. She is particularly popular with many of the residents' families. In this photograph, Carol talks with Pat on the day she placed her mother Hazel in the nursing home. Carol befriended Pat and helped her realize she had made the best decision.

I've been a professional aide for fourteen years and have worked here for three-and-a-half years. It takes a knack to be a nurse's aide. You can't pull somebody off the street and expect them to take care of people in bed who are incontinent, take care of backrubs, clean them up if they're sick to their stomach—anything like this. I work here on the North hall where most of the people get along by themselves. I take care of eighteen patients myself. Out of that I give backrubs, I give oral care, I feed them, I get them ready for bed, I pick up meal trays, I answer lights all night, and I empty bedpans. It's not an easy job. It's not always a pleasant job.

Good aides are hard to come by—the ones that really care about the residents, the ones that are able to take some abuse from the residents. Some of the kids think that they're the only ones who can get mad and blow up. They think that the residents are supposed to be goody-two-shoes all the time. It's not that way. The old people have to release their hostility too, just like anybody else. One time we had to remove an impaction from one of the residents. I had hold of her hands and the next thing I knew she had my finger in her mouth and was biting just as hard as she could. After we finished, she looked up at me and said, "Honey, I just had to let somebody know how bad that hurt."

—Carol

ROSE

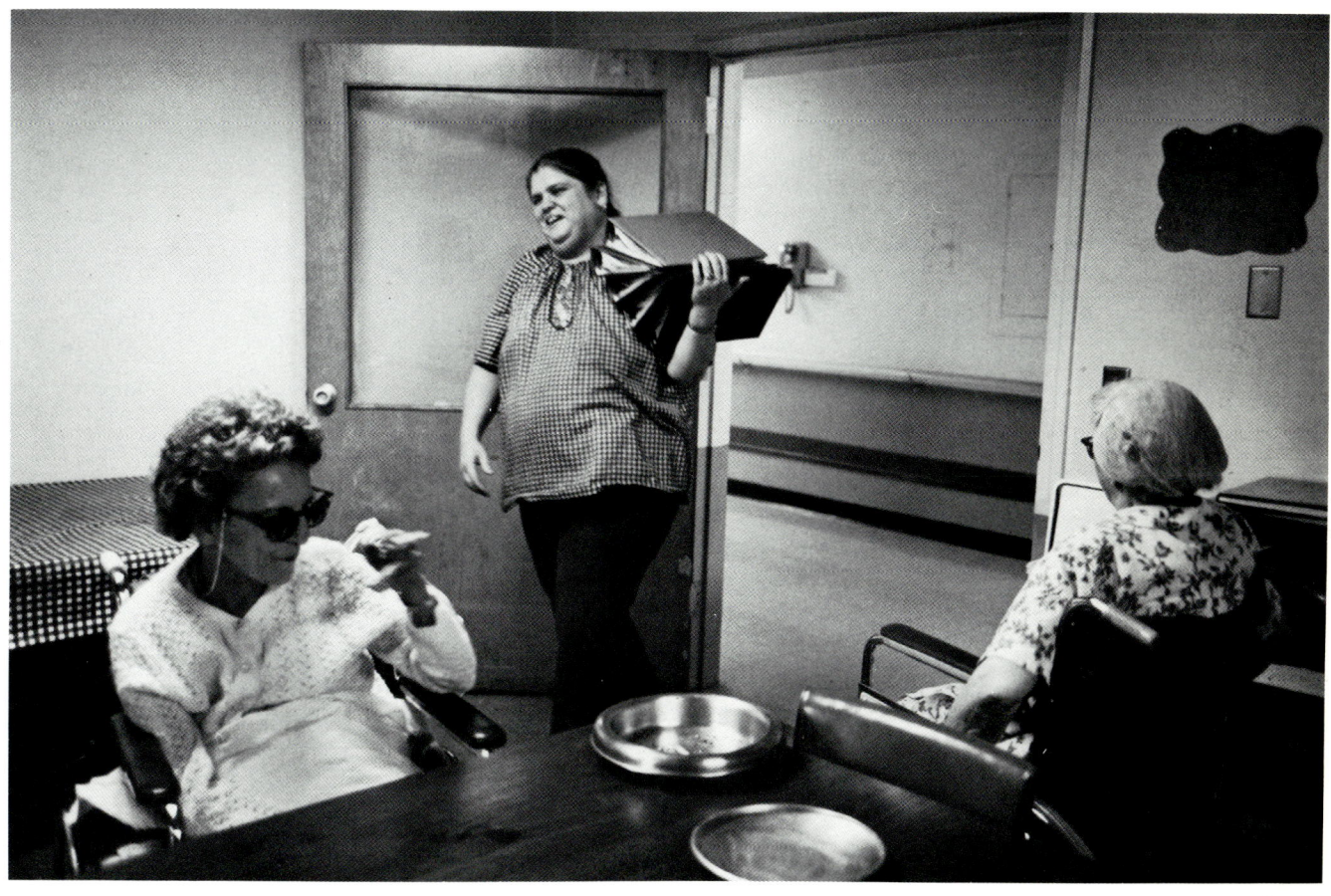

Two hours before her shift as an aide begins, Rose hangs out in the staff lounge munching on potato chips and reading a Harlequin romance. Frequently residents will come in to engage her in some lively banter. Or they hit her up for a Coke. They have learned she is an easy mark.

Rose is an enormously strong woman. When I worked as an aide, she would sneak up behind me, engage me in a massive bearhug, and in one clean jerk lift me off the floor as if I were a feather.

I'm fat and I'm jolly. The younger people call me names, but I get along well with the old people. Some of them got pet names for me. Alma calls me "The Little One." Wanda calls me "Teenie Weenie." A couple of them don't talk to me at all. I show my affection for them by putting my arm around them and giving them a big hug. They really enjoy it. There's a couple of them who don't mind the hugging part, but they don't want me to kiss them. They say women shouldn't kiss like that. But the guys really like it. There's a couple of them who've propositioned me to go to bed with 'em. I don't take them seriously, but I'll walk up to them and pester and tickle them.

Some of them act like little kids. Got to scold them once in a while. Like Archie. He really gets on my nerves. One night, I had to dress him five times. For my reward, I got kicked. I got literally kicked! I felt like giving him a hard slap, but I didn't. It's part of the job.

—Rose

ALICE

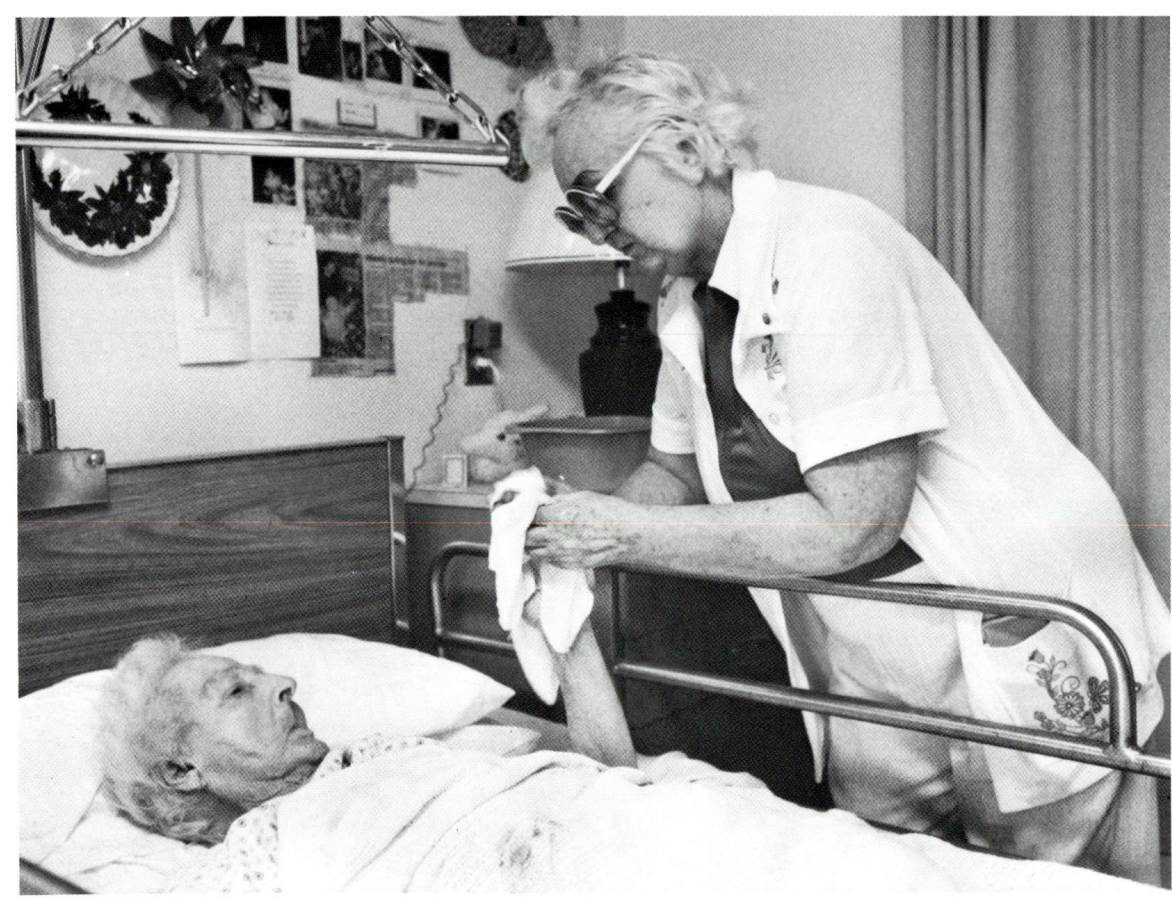

Alice, 65, has been a professional nurse's aide for over thirty years. She began working at the nursing home in the 1970s but was forced to retire five years later for health reasons. Within several months, Alice found she missed the work, so she returned and took a less physically demanding job delivering the residents personal laundry. Alice enjoys getting involved with the residents, bringing them candy and flowers, shopping for them, and even inviting them to her home for dinner.

When a resident dies, Alice observes the ritual of spending several minutes with the deceased. She and her friend Miriam always keep a careful eye on the morticians who come to claim the bodies to ensure that the deceased are accorded respect. On one occasion, Alice took one of the morticians to task for roughly handling a body. She then stood guard at the window. Just when the mortician was about to load the gurney into the hearse, she banged on the window. He looked toward Alice, then ever so gently guided the gurney inside.

We have patients who are very interesting and they have a lot of tales to tell us. Like the man who used to herd cattle. He used to sleep out at night under the stars watching the cattle—just like you read about in the cowboy stories. Then there was the lady who used to be a dancer in Vegas, and there was another one who was a concert pianist. One lady even trapped wolves in Alaska. But we have others who start to tell you something and they flake out on you; they can't remember. Then there are the cynics who don't want to know anything. Some residents try to keep going, try to stay alert by watching TV and reading, but others will simply get up in the morning and just stare at the wall. Now they could do better, they could help themselves, but they're not interested. Like we had a patient who came in here about six months ago and told us straight off the bat that she had come here to die. She said that her people had put her in here, and that she was going to die. She wouldn't eat, she wouldn't do anything. And honest to God, within two-and-a-half weeks she was dead.

—Alice

TWENTY-TWO TIMES

I've worked here off and on for about five years and my Mom has worked here for almost seven years. I left a while back to go to work at Guardian Photo. There I was sitting on my butt all day sending out photos and it was boring. I got fired 'cause I was too slow, so I came back here because I knew there would be an opening. At Guardian you never had a chance to know your co-workers, but here you're always helping each other out.

I always asked Mom for help when I first started working here. I really look up to her. Mom is one of those people you can always depend on. Even if it's raining, sleeting, or snowing, she'll come to work. But I won't bring myself to the level of having her as my own ego. If I did, Mom would hate my guts. She told me not to look up to her as my superior and after I got to know my job I saw her as another aide. Yet there are days when we cry on each other's shoulders. Two weeks ago one of my patients had diarrhea twenty-two times, and I was so upset. Besides that I wasn't feeling well. I said to myself, "I wish Mom was here," but she was on the other side giving showers. The charge nurse finally sent over a couple of girls to help me get caught up and one of them was Mom. I cried on her shoulders for five minutes. "Shirley, what are you doing?" she asked. "It's been one of those days," I told her. "It isn't that bad," she said. "But twenty-two times!" I said. Then we both started laughing.

There are days when Mom needs help, too. I'll ask the other aides to keep an eye on her. I don't want her to overwork herself. Some of the aides will take advantage of her by having Mom do their work. One of these days I'll punch one of them in the mouth.

With the years creeping up on Mom, I find it really difficult to think about sending her to a nursing home. Our love for each other is really something. I think I would end up taking care of her, rather than send her to a nursing home. It's not because of the care she would get—it's pretty good. But some of the aides they hire are pretty bad. I just couldn't stand to see my Mom mistreated.

I don't want to be an aide for a lifetime career like my mother did. Mom is good at her work and has been a professional aide for over twenty years. I'm proud to say that she is really an excellent aide. I'm not saying that I'm not a good aide, but I don't want this to be my lifetime career. I'm still young and there are other things and other places out there for me to experience. But for a while, I'll do it.

—Shirley

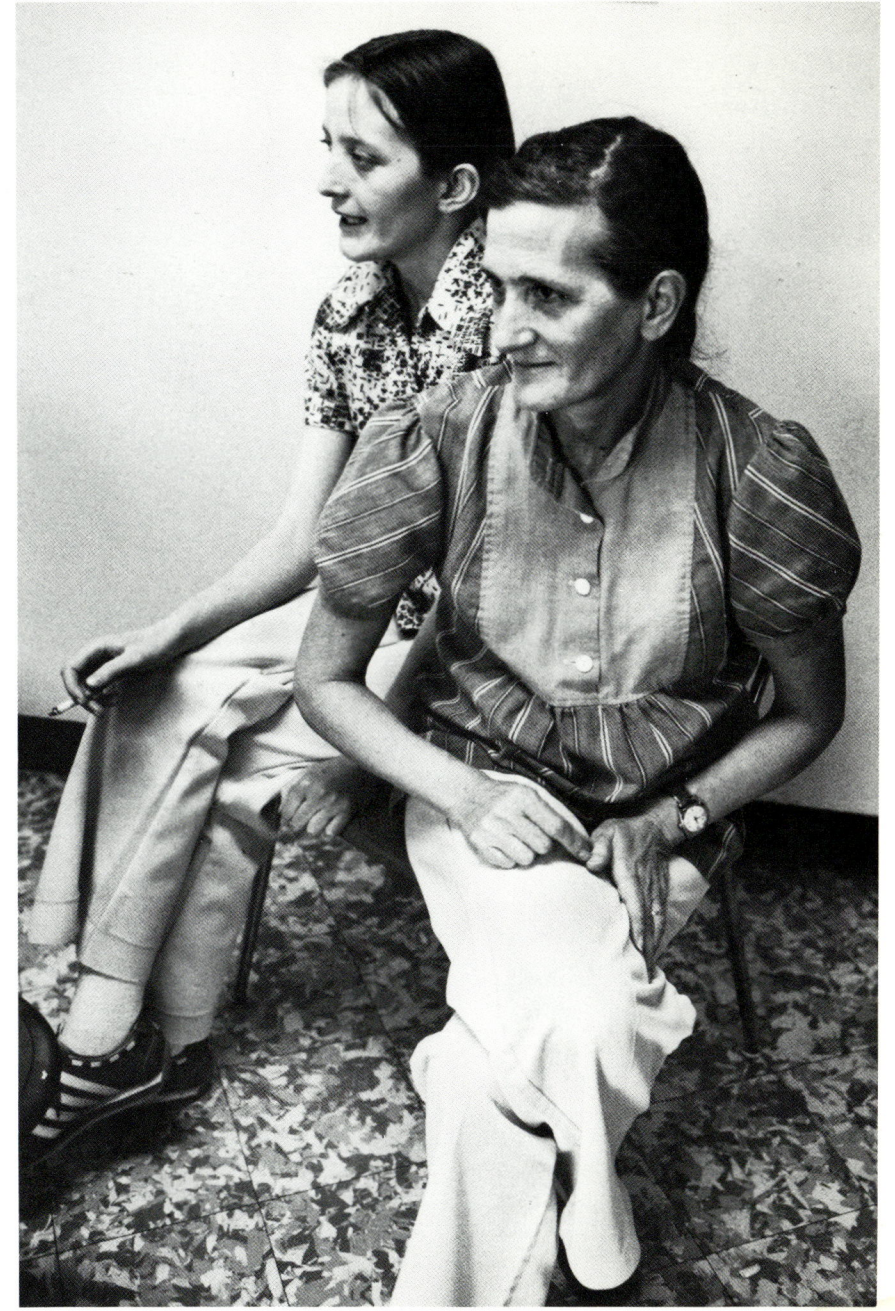

IV. Outsiders

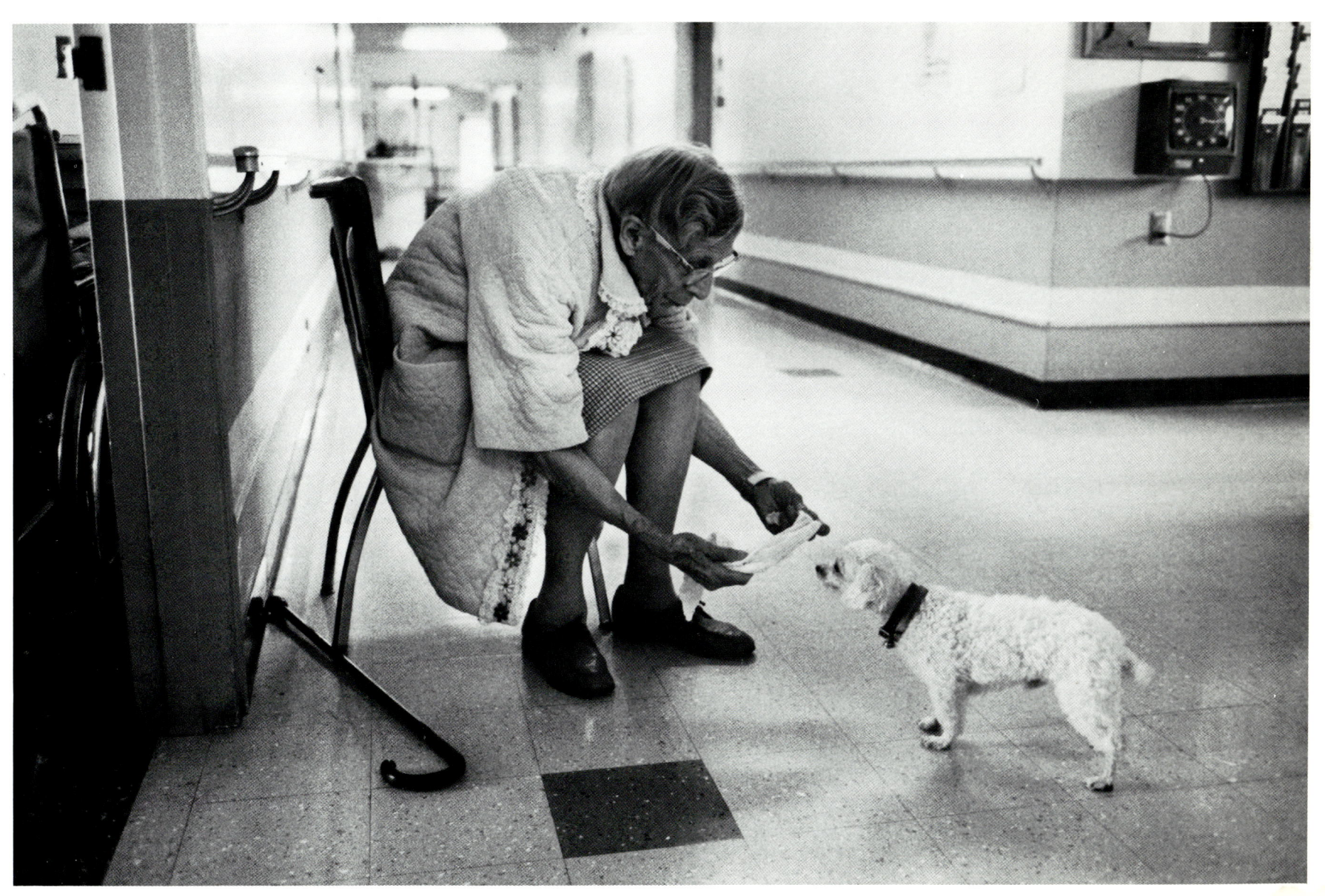

TELEVISION

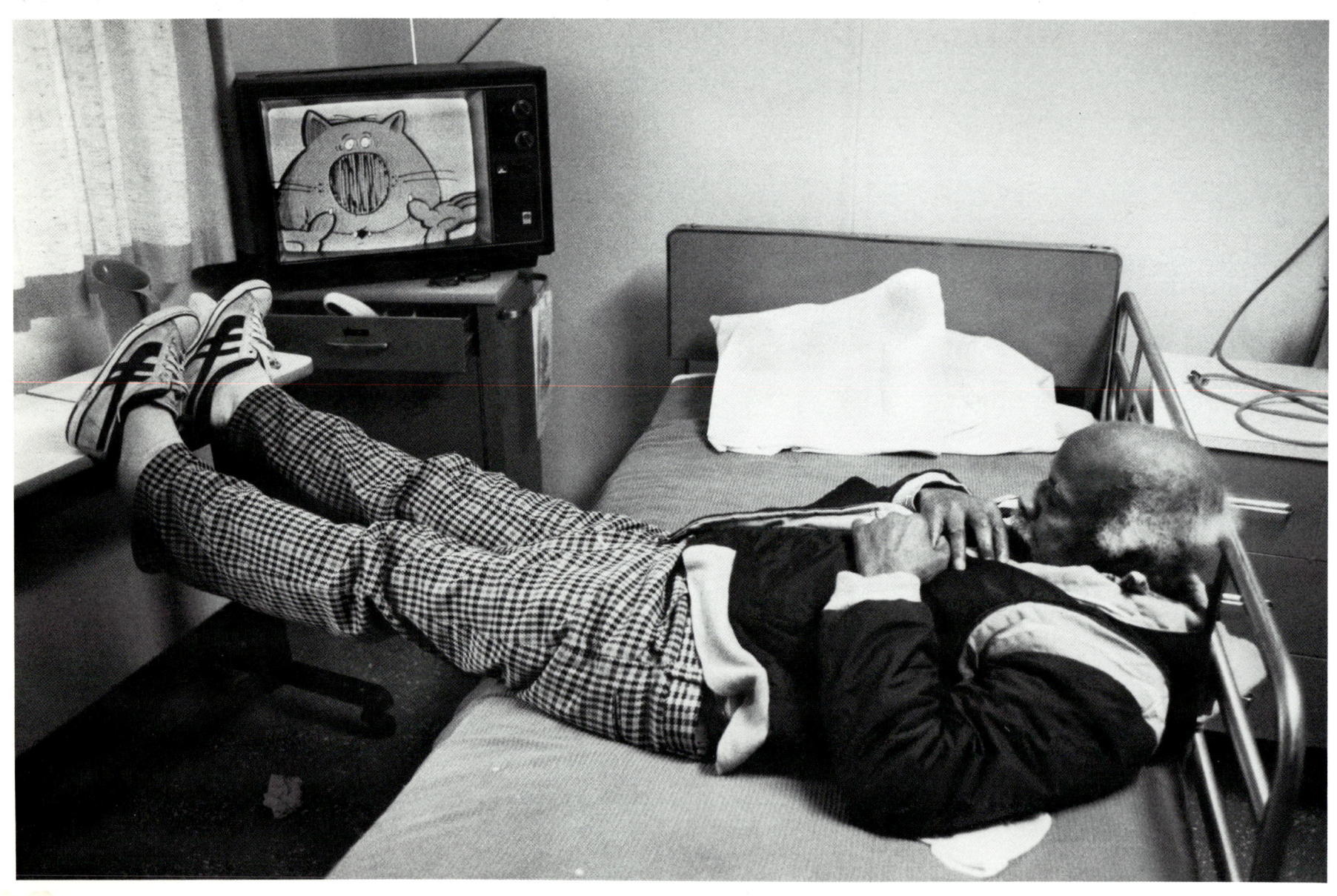

SANTA CLAUS

I felt like a nut when Santa Claus came up to me and kissed me. I thought it was out of place. Old people don't have a need for Santa Claus. But you can't be rude to people like that—maybe she was having a good time. She should have paid more attention to the children than the old people. Maybe she thinks we are all senile and don't know what we're doing. But I still have my faculties. Just 'cause I don't have any legs and am a little old woman—that doesn't excuse her.

—Georgia

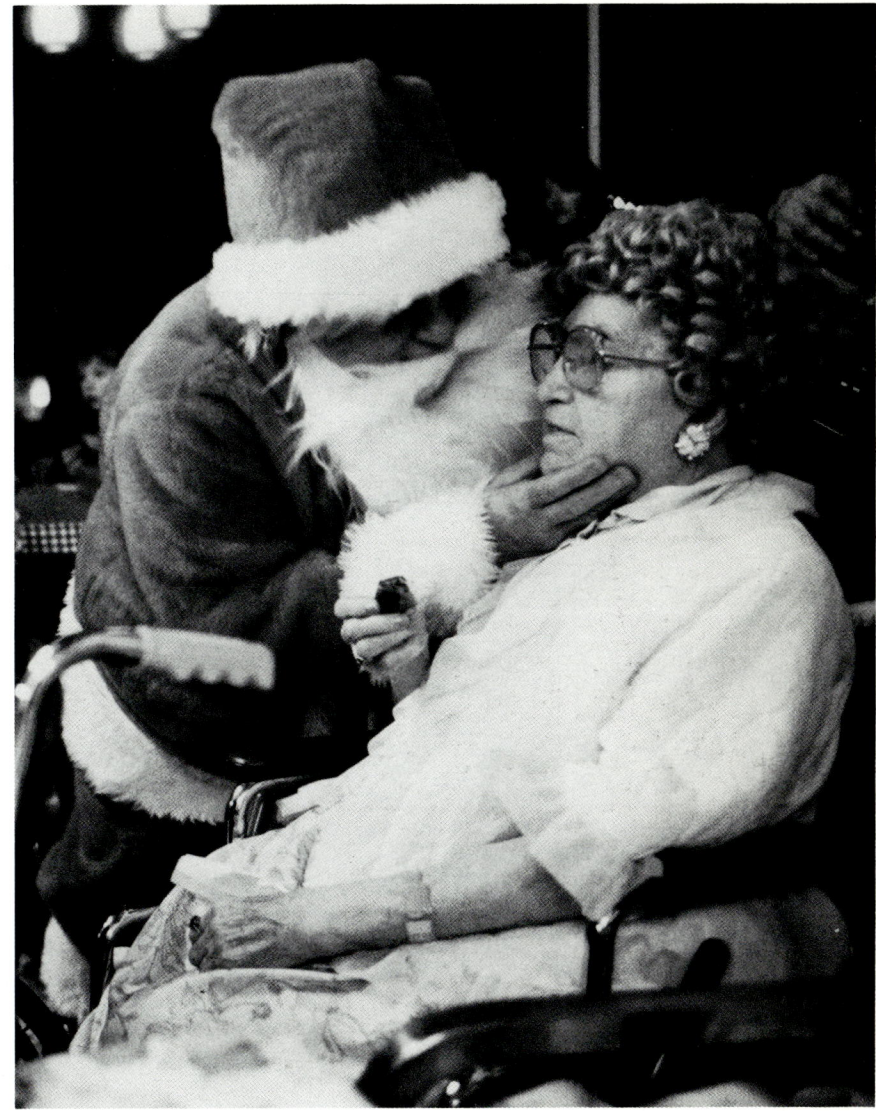

SENIOR PRODUCER, TOWN HALL

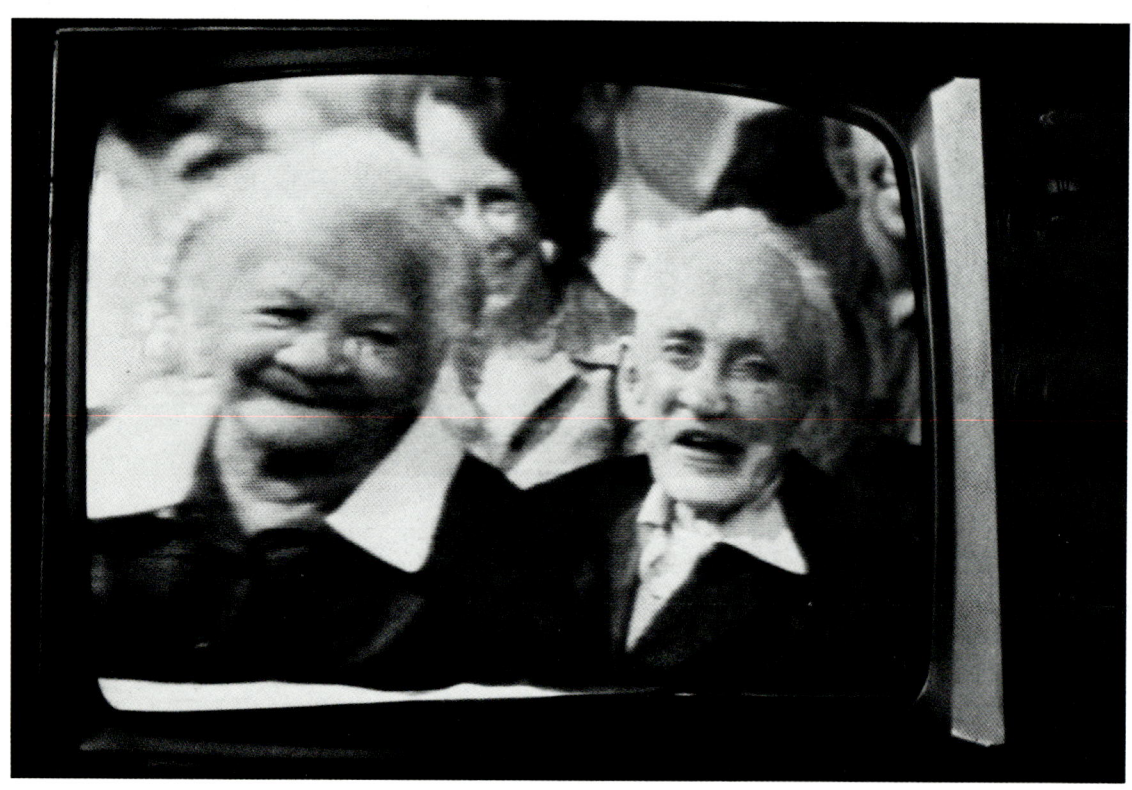

Town Hall, a weekly, hour-long television program reminiscent of the old-time town meeting, has a moderator and community members as participating audience. When it was decided to present "The Hell of Growing Old," Lisa, the senior producer, and her staff spent a week at the nursing home preparing for the show.

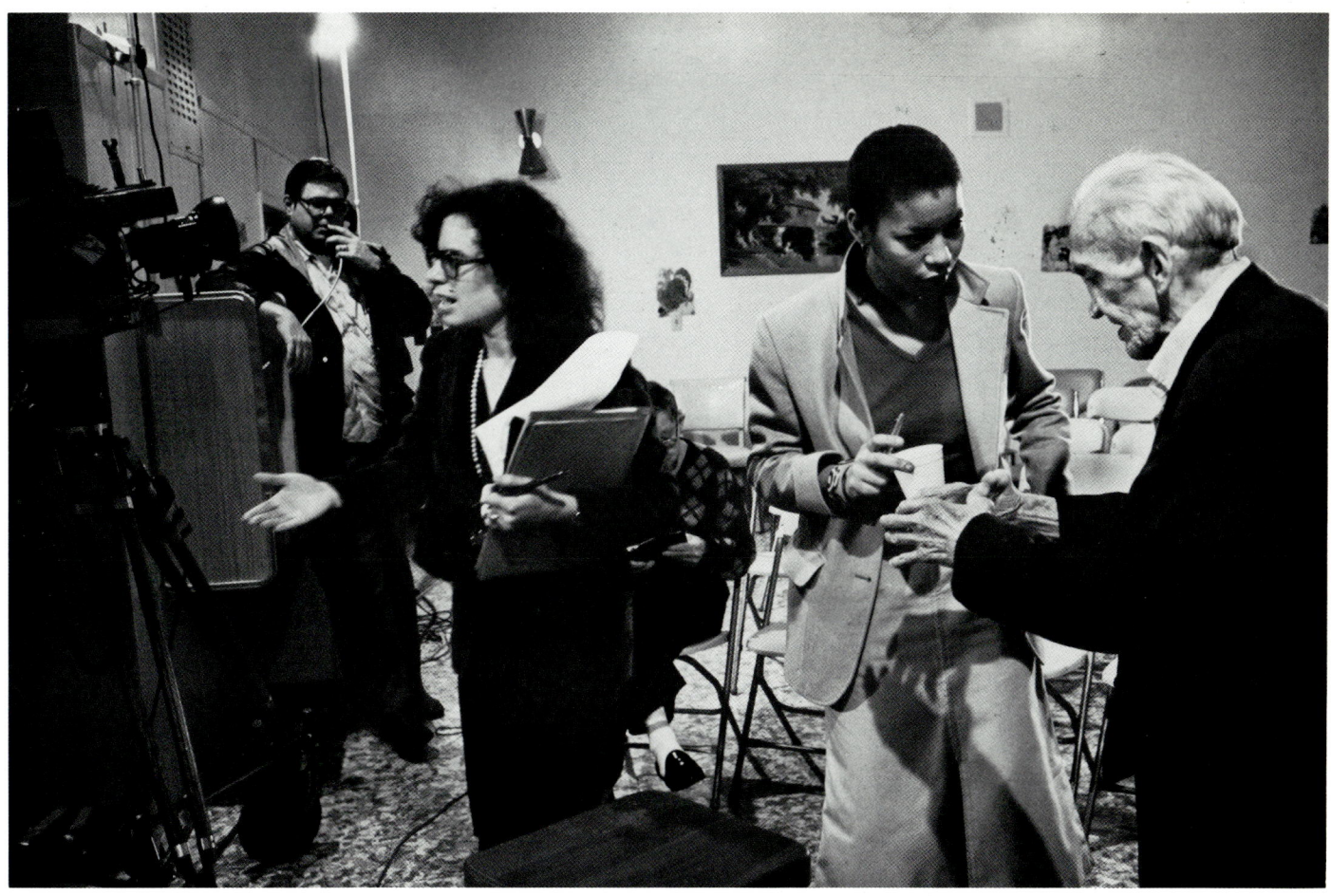

I'm the senior producer from Town Hall. I've never been in a nursing home before, so it's very tough emotionally for me to be here. I think it's a depressing experience for anyone who isn't used to it. In these situations, you always reflect yourself in a mirror—in fifty years this could be you and probably will be you.

In some respects, the nursing home is like a prison; it's an institution for those who can't care for themselves. A lot of people lose their self-respect, their dignity. As we went through the home with our cameras, no one stopped us from going into the residents' rooms. People just seemed resigned to the lack of privacy. What I found most depressing were the cards and photographs on the walls that some residents couldn't remember anymore.

I hope the residents open up and talk about some of their problems. Hopefully, people will realize that they're not all senile, that they do have something to say, and that they care about what is going on in the world. It's going to be a difficult show. The public thinks that nursing home residents have lost contact with reality. After spending a week here myself, I discovered that it isn't necessarily true. I really warmed up to the people.

—Lisa

FATHER HOWARD

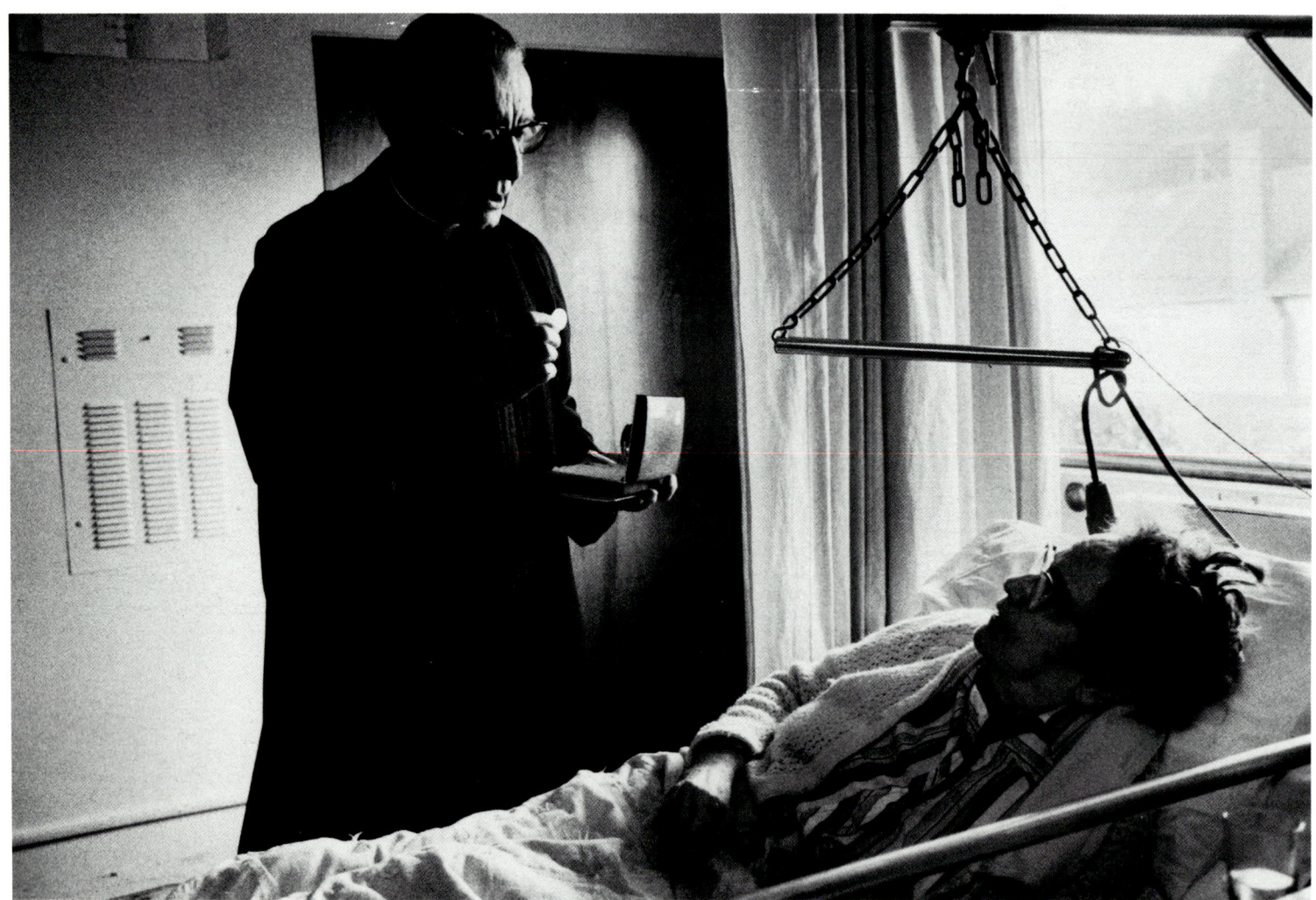

I'm seventy-one, and I've been seeing residents who are in our own parish as well as those who belong to other parishes. There is a real need for someone like myself to visit them. Anybody can end up in a place like this. It gives me courage to see residents who are suffering well. You can learn a lot from them. You learn to accept God's will.

FUNERAL DIRECTOR

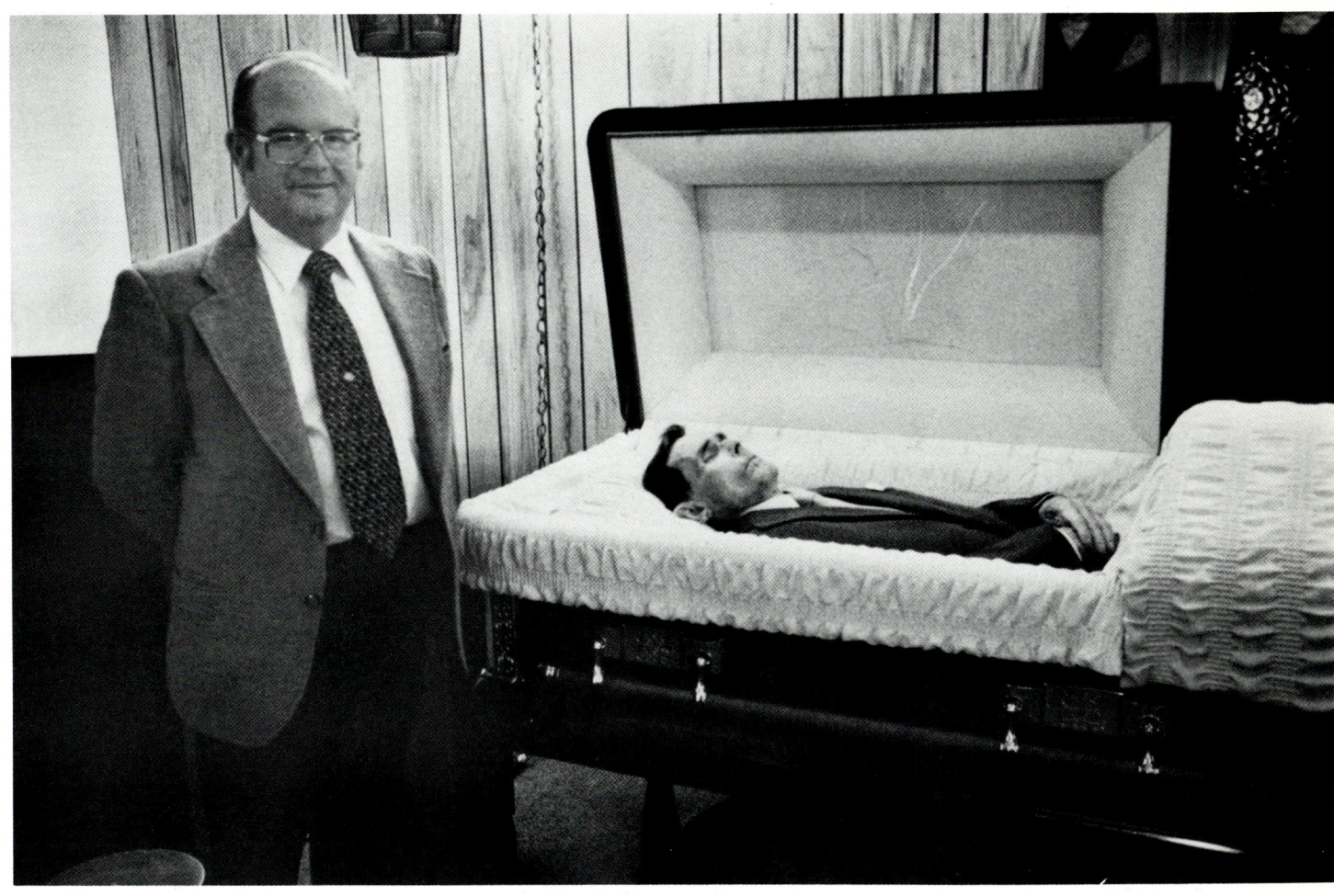

When Leroy, a resident at the nursing home, died, his funeral was held at a small neighborhood mortuary that has been in business over seventy-five years. The Vice President of the home handled the funeral arrangements.

Leroy's stepmother, who played the organ during the service, recalls, " 'Until Then' was one of the hymns I thought he would love. That was one of the hymns played at my brother's funeral three years ago." Leroy had a proper sendoff. All of the family attended his funeral.

Many younger people who come to funerals no longer wear black suits. They come in jeans. These kids are the death deniers. They'll sit in my office while I'm making funeral arrangements for their parents or grandparents, and to them the whole thing is very absurd. I'll ask the family, "Would you like a soloist?" The kids will look up at the ceiling and roll their eyes in the back of their heads like, Oh my God, you got to be kidding, they're going to sing hymns. I feel like saying, "Why don't you sit there and be quiet, and see what happens before you pass judgment?" After the funeral, many of these kids really appreciate how much we've done for them and the rest of the family. You really feel good about it. If you didn't have these good feelings, this would be a lousy business.

—Dan

BROTHER LOREN

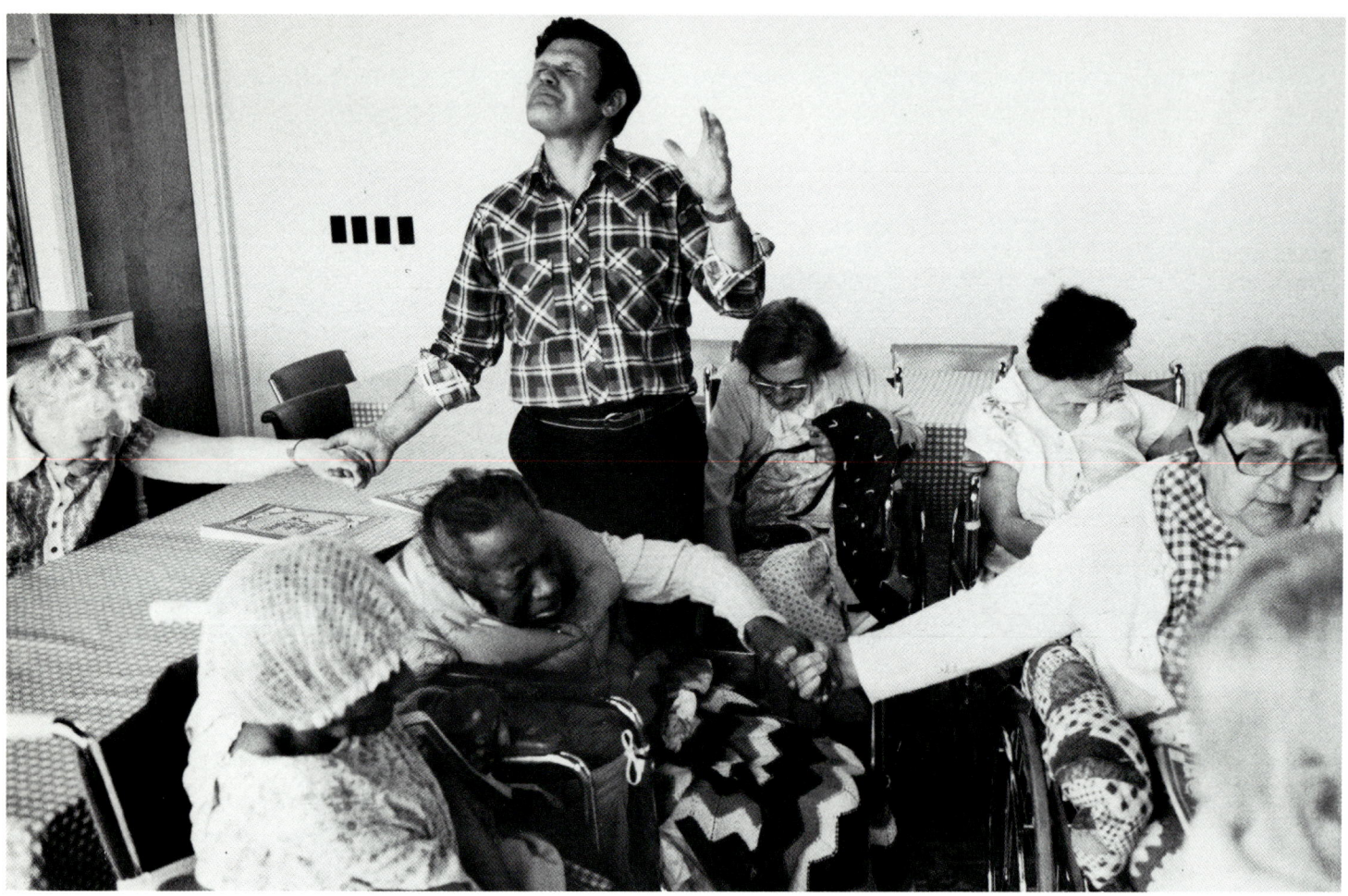

Every Saturday afternoon around 2:30, the powerful voice of Brother Loren, a lay preacher, booms from the North dining room. The place is hot and moist with religion. He reads from the Bible, preaches, leads gathered residents in song, and invites them to give personal testimony on the goodness of the Lord. Brother Loren is well-liked by his congregation, and unlike many of the other evangelicals that come to the nursing home, he personally knows everybody in his congregation.

I got saved in 1950, and not too long after that I started preaching. In those days when a person got saved the most natural thing in the world to do was to go out into the streets and witness, so I witnessed in carnivals, on skid row, and even did just plain street work, witnessing and handing out tracts.

Of all my different ministries the nursing home took the most training. My initial reaction was one of fear. I really didn't understand how to approach old people. At first I tried to avoid anything that would be painful, like talking about death, because they were so close to it, because so many of them were dying. But I find that it is important to talk about death, to let them know that they are only falling asleep in Jesus.

They are all special, but there was this one dear old lady who was a hundred years old and really perky. She couldn't hear, but she would sit up real close and cup her ear, and I would talk real loud. Then she would give testimony, about the goodness of the Lord and what the Lord had done for her. She was alive, totally alive, unto the Lord. One day she fell, and after that she became disoriented, but every time I would talk about the Lord she would snap right out of it. She used to say "Open up those gates wide, I want to come home." She was so tired and so ready to go home. I miss her terribly at times—but at the same time, the peace.

The thing that I hear that is really the most heartbreaking to me is, "I have to be here and I want to be home. My family betrayed me by putting me in here." One lady said, "Do you mean I've got to be happy here? I refuse to be happy as long as I have to be here." She refused to be comforted is what it came right down to. This is the hardest thing, trying to comfort someone who has a crippled spirit. I can see crippled bodies, I can see sickness, and I can see all those things, but the thing that drains me more than anything else is the mental anguish of the people.

If I get down, I can go for a walk, and be alone and pray. It seems that if I had these same emotional problems, these same doubts, and I was trapped in bed and couldn't even go out for a walk, the depression and melancholy would be so much more severe. What is required in a situation like this is more confidence through spiritual awareness. And this is what I try to work with, confidence in a God who has everything under control.

—Brother Loren

V. Reflections

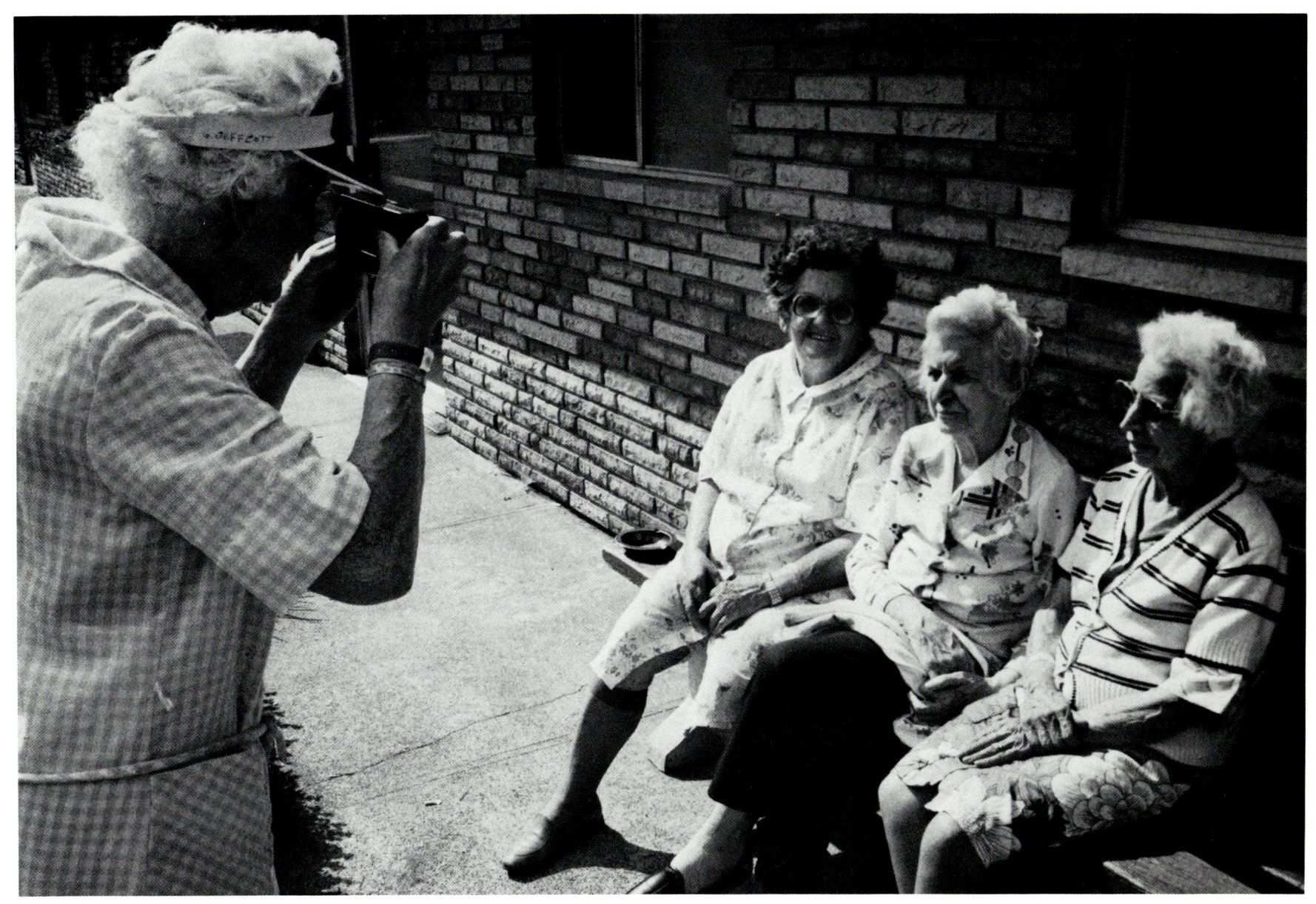

FLYING EAST

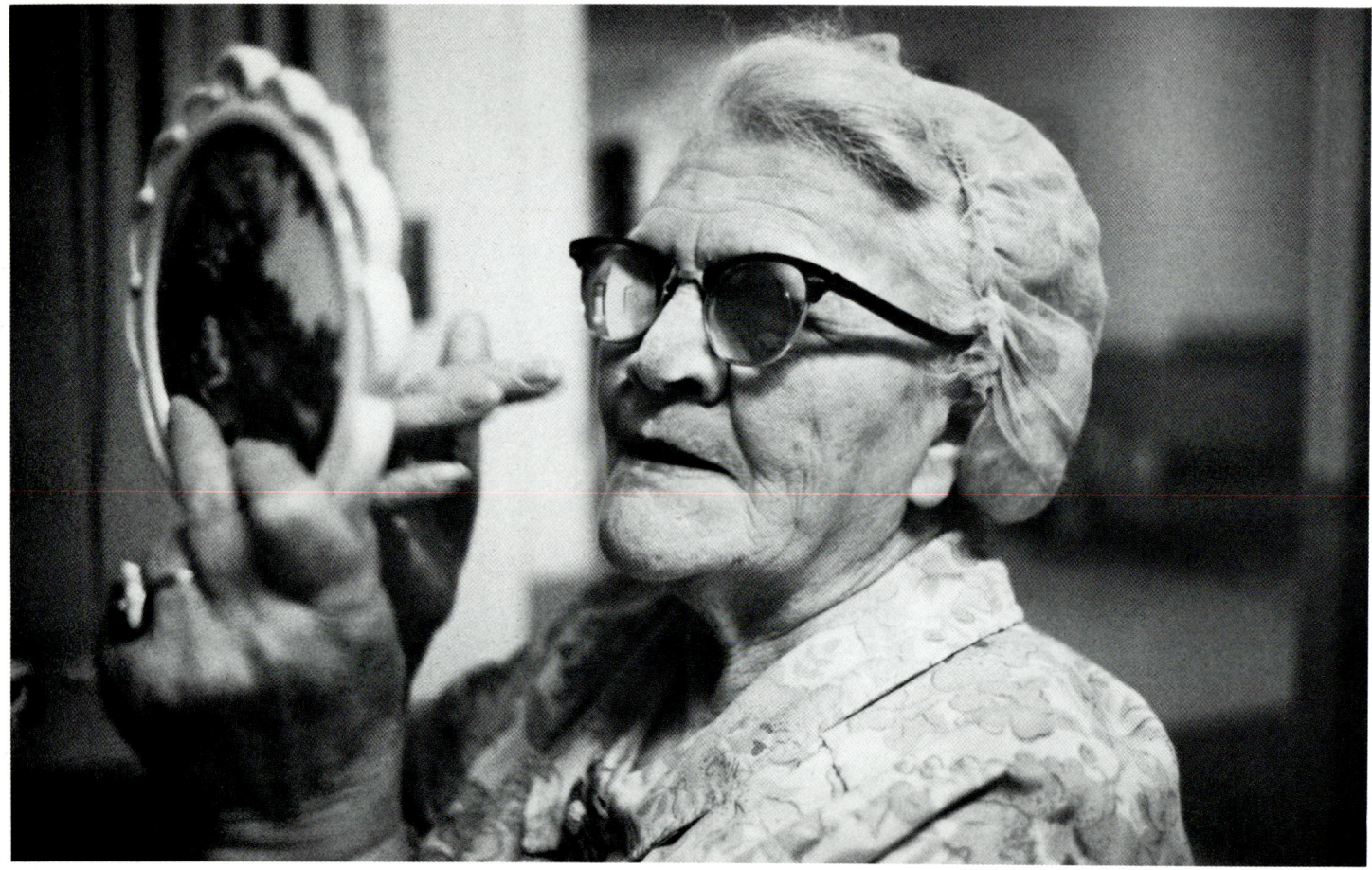

I have the craziest dreams. I dreamed about goin' back to Iowa where I was born. I'm flying East, over the Great Lakes, and I finally land at Ferguson, Iowa, where I was born. So many of my family are gone now. My mother and father, of course. My younger brother got killed in a construction accident. My son, who was an officer in the Navy, got mugged in Long Beach, California. Someone hit him on the head and he died of head injuries. When I'm tired and restless, I'll have the craziest dreams.

—Frances

HE WAS A GOOD MAN

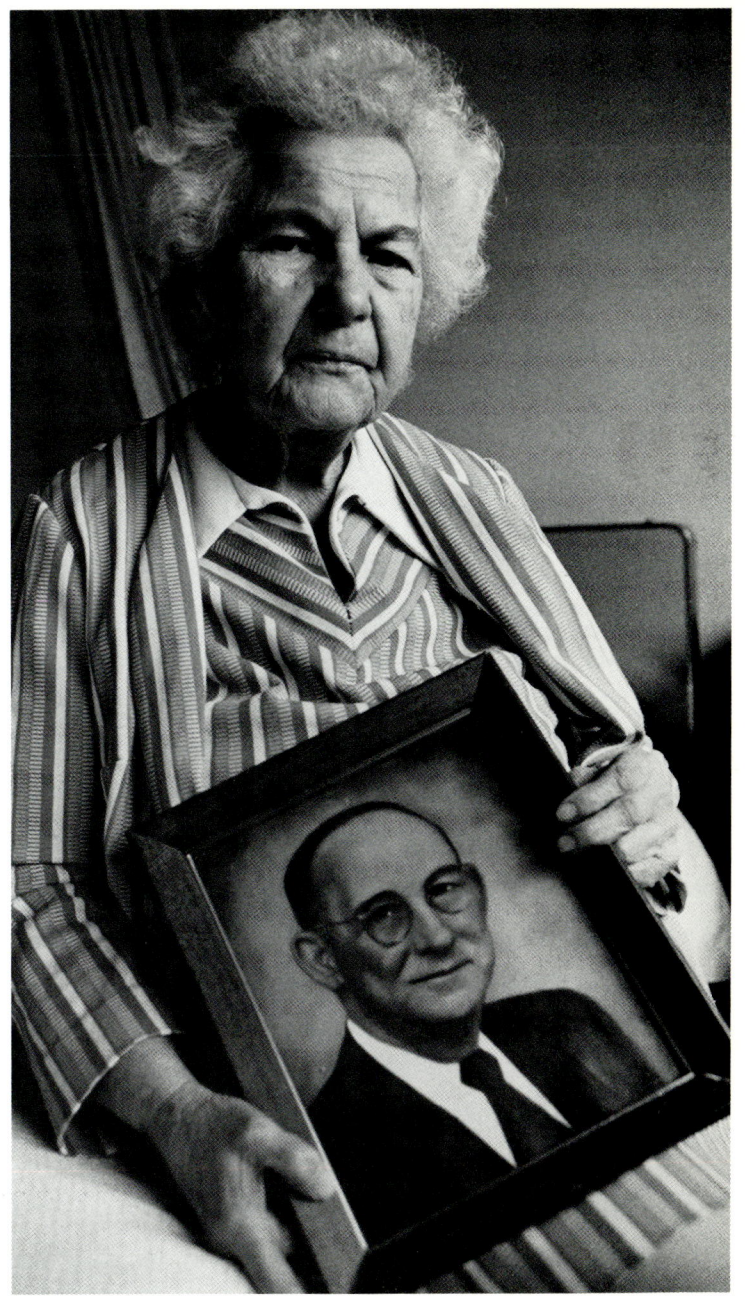

—Ruby, with a portrait of her husband.

HORATIO

I used to be a dancer in China and Japan. I had my own show. I was with my second husband, Orville D. Harder, at the time, and he was a great manager. He named the show after me, and everywhere we went, we were invited to go to other places.

I remember when we were in Shanghai, and we wanted to go to Shing-shin to do a show. It wasn't Shing-shin, it was . . . I can't imagine me forgetting these things. Anyway, in this town there was no place where people could go. They had no theaters, not even saloons, and the people didn't know what to do to amuse themselves. So I talked to a Chinaman, a wealthy Chinaman, and asked him if he'd like to build up a show business there. He said he would. He said he wanted something swell, something like America had.

He had a big park built, and he bought a showhouse and fixed it up. Then he advertised me: Ramona in a great new dance with a big snake. And I mean it was a great big snake. The Chinaman owned it, and its name was Horatio. I didn't mind snakes—I could handle 'em. But on opening night, my husband was playing with Horatio, had him wrapped around his waist, and when they tried to take the snake off of him, Horatio wouldn't let go. It took four fellas to pull that snake off. The Chinaman didn't think I should use Horatio in my act. He was afraid it might kill me. So I put the show on alone.

—Ramona

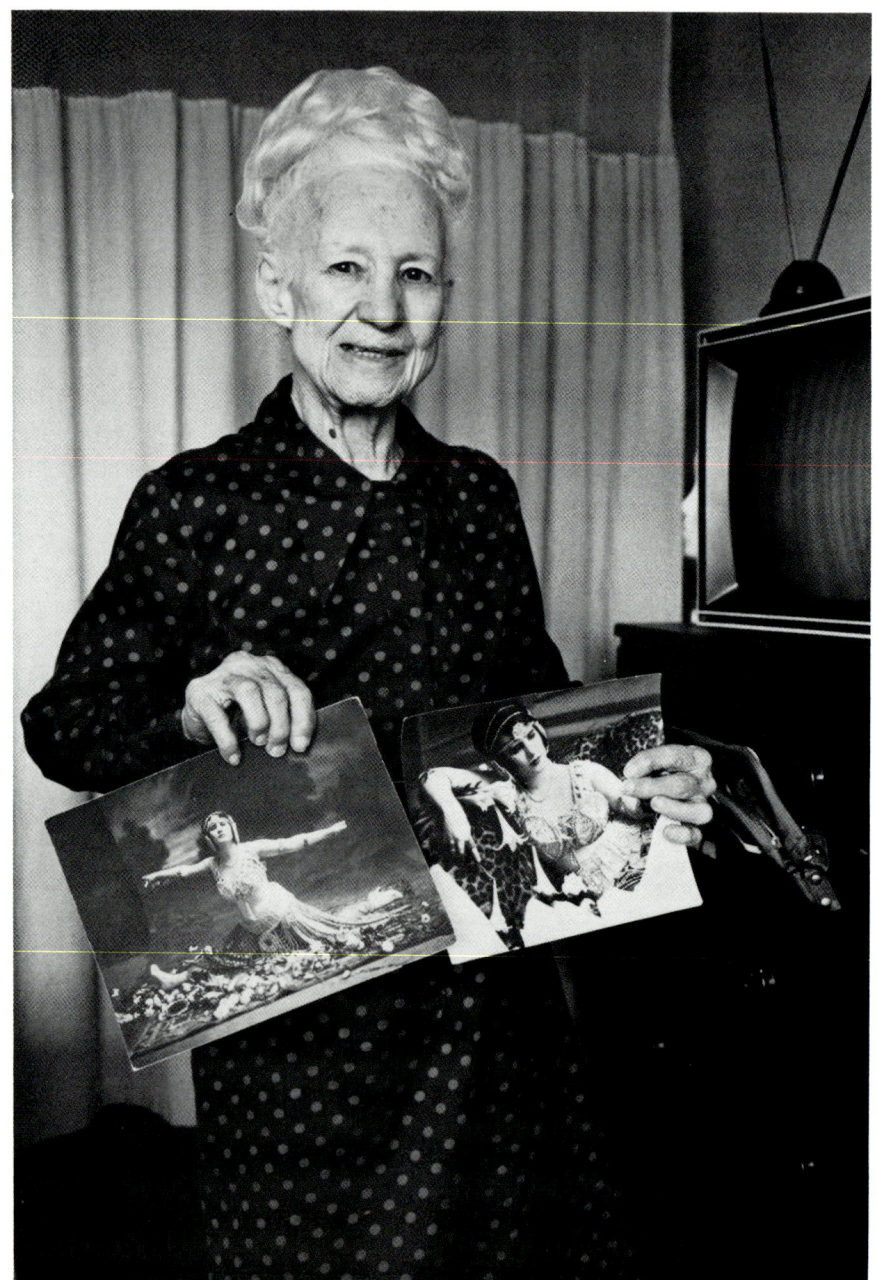

NOBODY LEFT

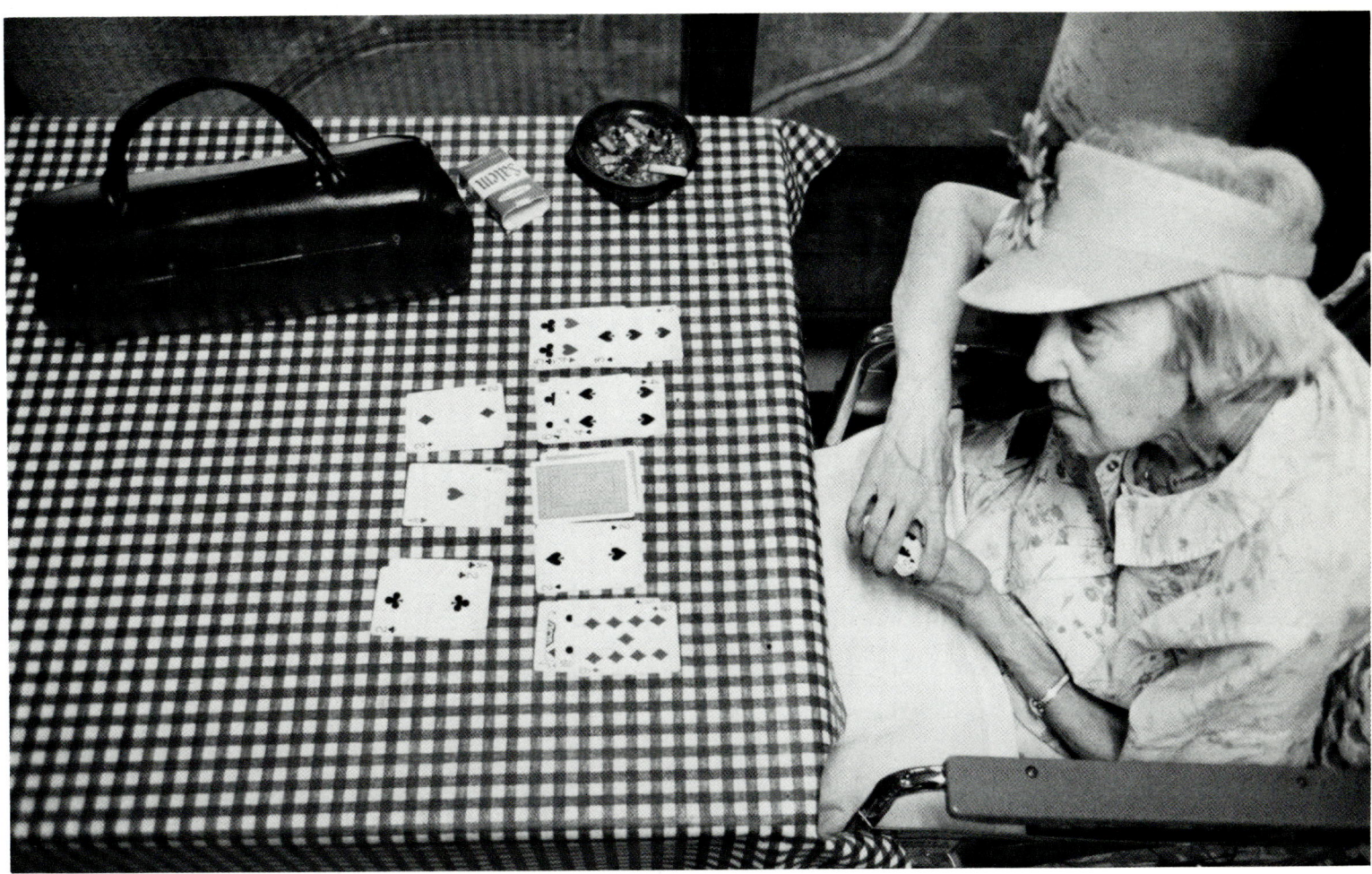

My first husband was killed in a dentist's chair. They didn't clap his tongue down and he choked to death on his own tongue. A friend of mine, old Doctor Apple, went to the autopsy . . . I asked him to. He said, "Ruth, they killed him." Nineteen thirty-seven, the T. W. Anderson Memorial Building. I've been thinking about that forty years. I live with it. And after my daughter was murdered I had a double wound. She was murdered in 1977. She left her husband and he didn't like it. And they're all my hell and all my heaven right here on earth. It's been a lot of hell. After my daughter's murder I was lost, sunk. My little four-pound baby girl. Now there isn't any life; I just exist. Where is your life in a place like this, or any other nursing home? Nobody left in the world you love. You can have it. I have some happy memories, but I have more unhappy ones than I do happy ones.

—Ruth

A TRAILER HOUSE IN THE COUNTRY

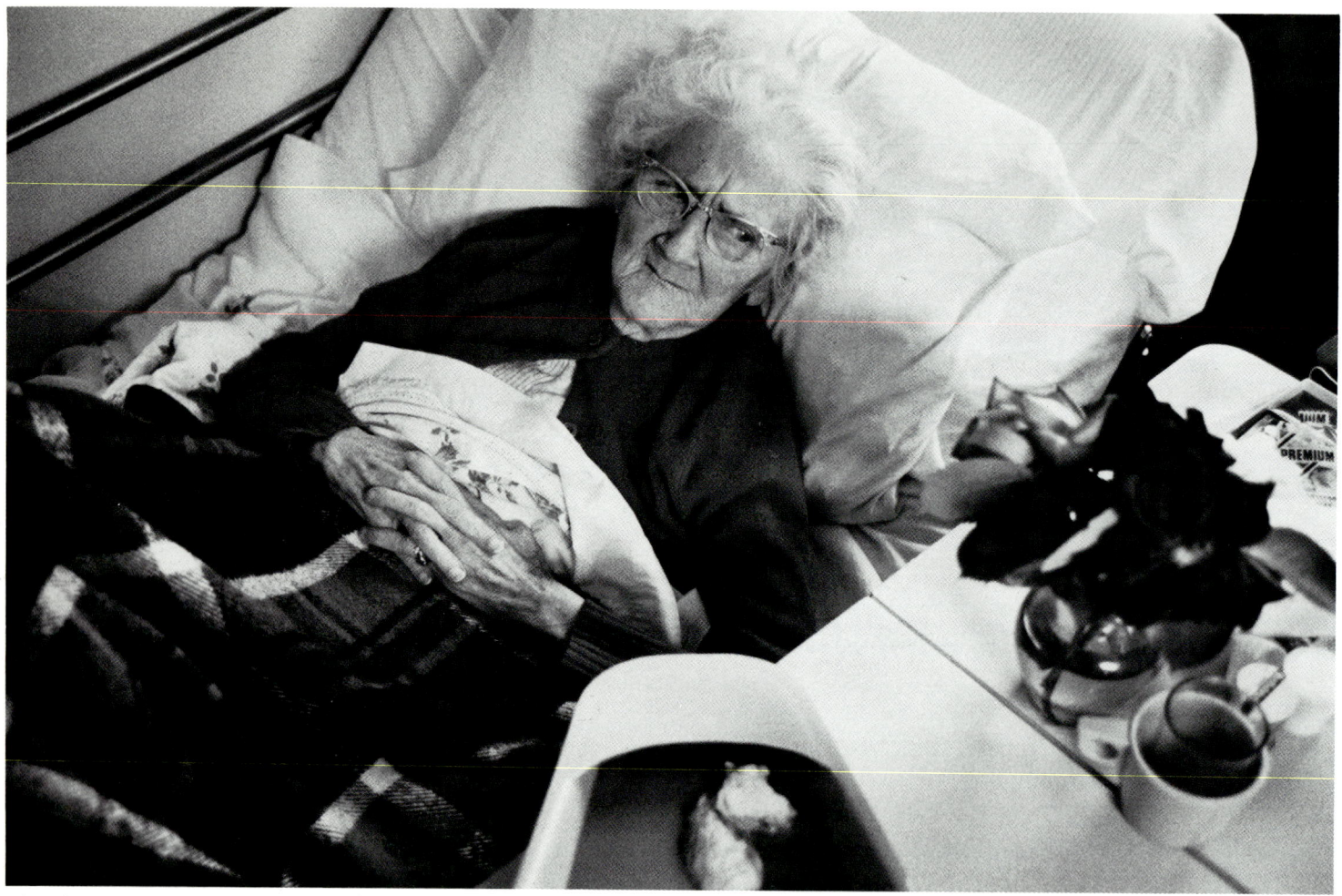

My dream is to have a trailer house in the country like I had when my husband was alive. Three rooms and a bath, new curtains, and a nice yard with lots of pretty flowers. I don't really care where it is as long as it's somewhere in the country. I'd be better off if I was out of this place. It doesn't get better, it gets worse.

My husband and I used to joke about who would be buried first in the Veterans' graveyard. We have a double grave. "Don't kid yourself," I told him, "you're going to be on the bottom." "Oh no I'm not," he said, "I'm going to be on top!" Well it turns out that I'm going to be on top and he is on the bottom. Sometimes I wish I was on the bottom.

—Minnie

I GOT PLENTY TO EAT

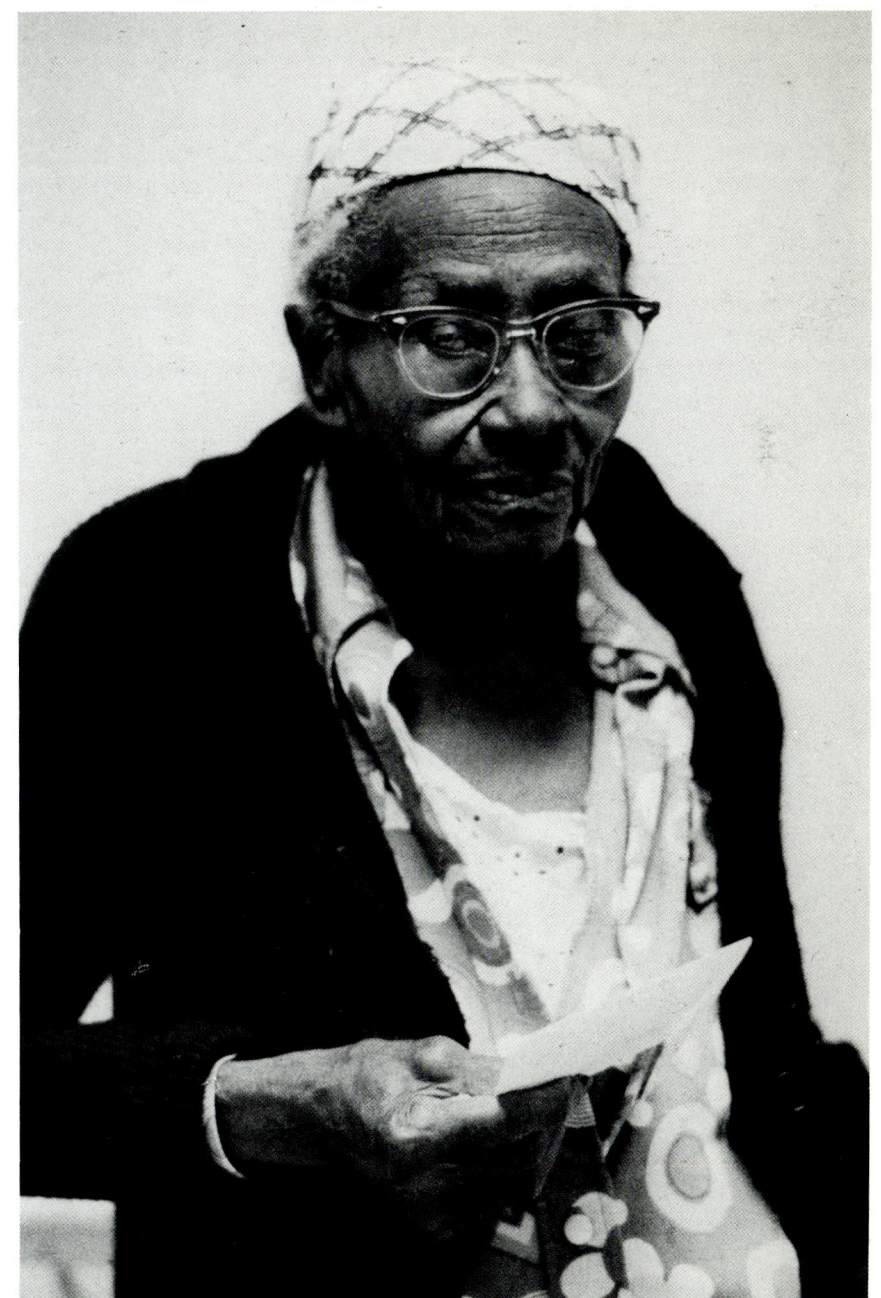

Are the Negroes getting their share? I'm getting mine but are the other people getting theirs? Some of them are complaining that they're not getting enough food. I'm getting enough, but I'm concerned about 'em. I've been through the same thing: not getting enough to eat. I've been in that shape so many times. Are they getting their share? Used to be that the white people got their share and the Negroes nothing. That's all over, for the government has taken care of it. I got plenty to eat.

—Phenie

WOMEN GET PUSHED AROUND

I don't run over anyone and I don't let anyone run over me. I'm not afraid to speak my mind. Some people are though, especially women. Women get pushed around. I've seen it, even here in the nursing home. I've worked for a good number of years and they expected more out of me than a man who did the same kind of work. As a woman, you get pushed around quite easily. I've started feeling this way since I've gotten older.

—Muriel

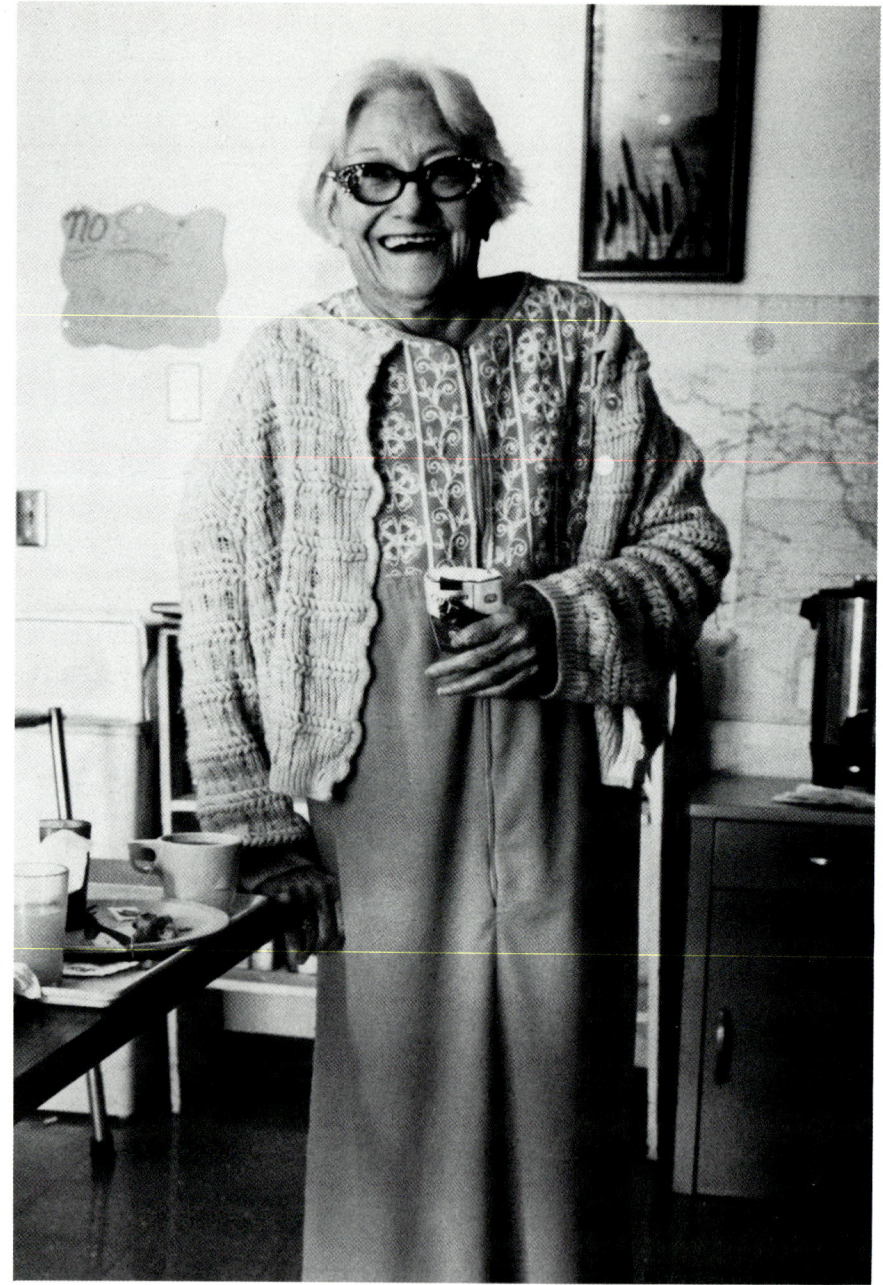

HERDING CATTLE

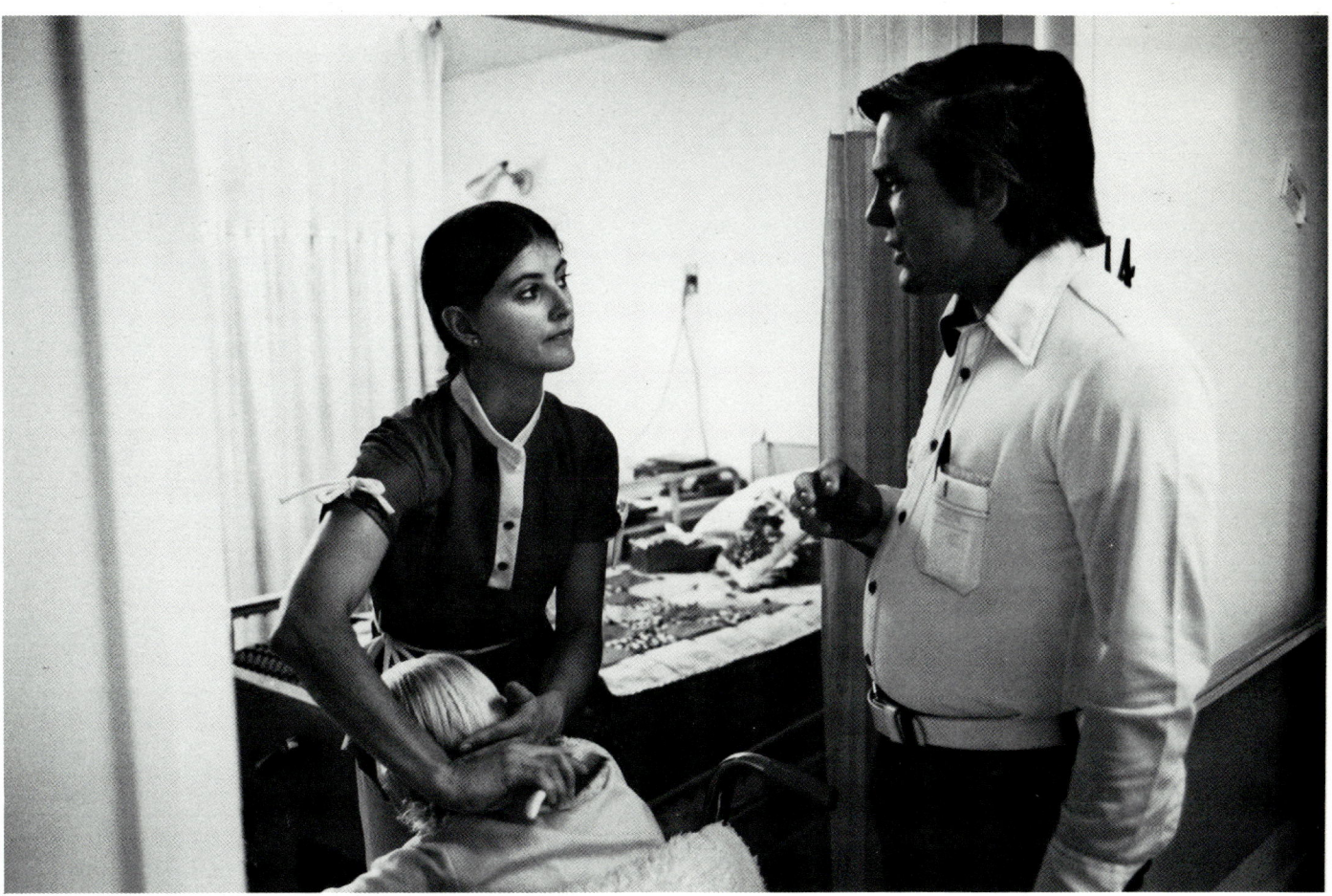

Since working here, I've noticed every time an aide brings up an idea nothing is ever done. Also, everything is so disorganized. We're always short of help. In the mornings when you give showers, you have to run patients in so fast you feel like you're herding cattle. It makes the girls so mad. In my opinion, we should get paid a lot more than we do. A lot of people look at us aides as if we are peons. There are not too many men who would be willing to do this work. So we started our organization.

The main goal that we are trying to accomplish is to get enough staff and get everyone to work together so that the residents get better care. Also, we are trying to get better wages. A lot of the girls are afraid to speak up about what makes them mad. But I'm not. That's why most of the girls elected me to be a head of our organization. When there is a problem I go right to the administration.

—Paula

HELL OF A BEAUTIFUL WOMAN

Ethel and I have always been great friends. I've known her for over forty-five years. She used to be one hell of a beautiful woman. She and my mother would go into the butcher shop and she would smile, and the poor butcher would start throwing the meat around without looking.

—Bill

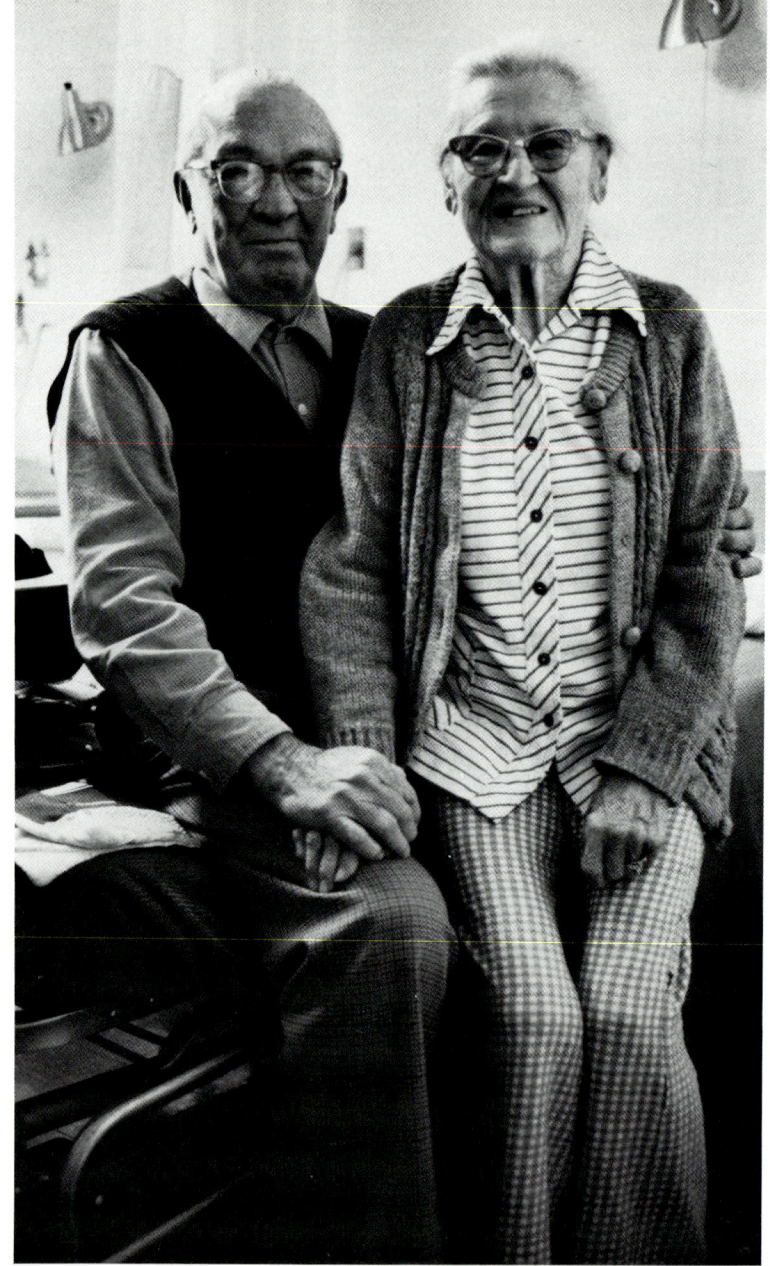

BABY

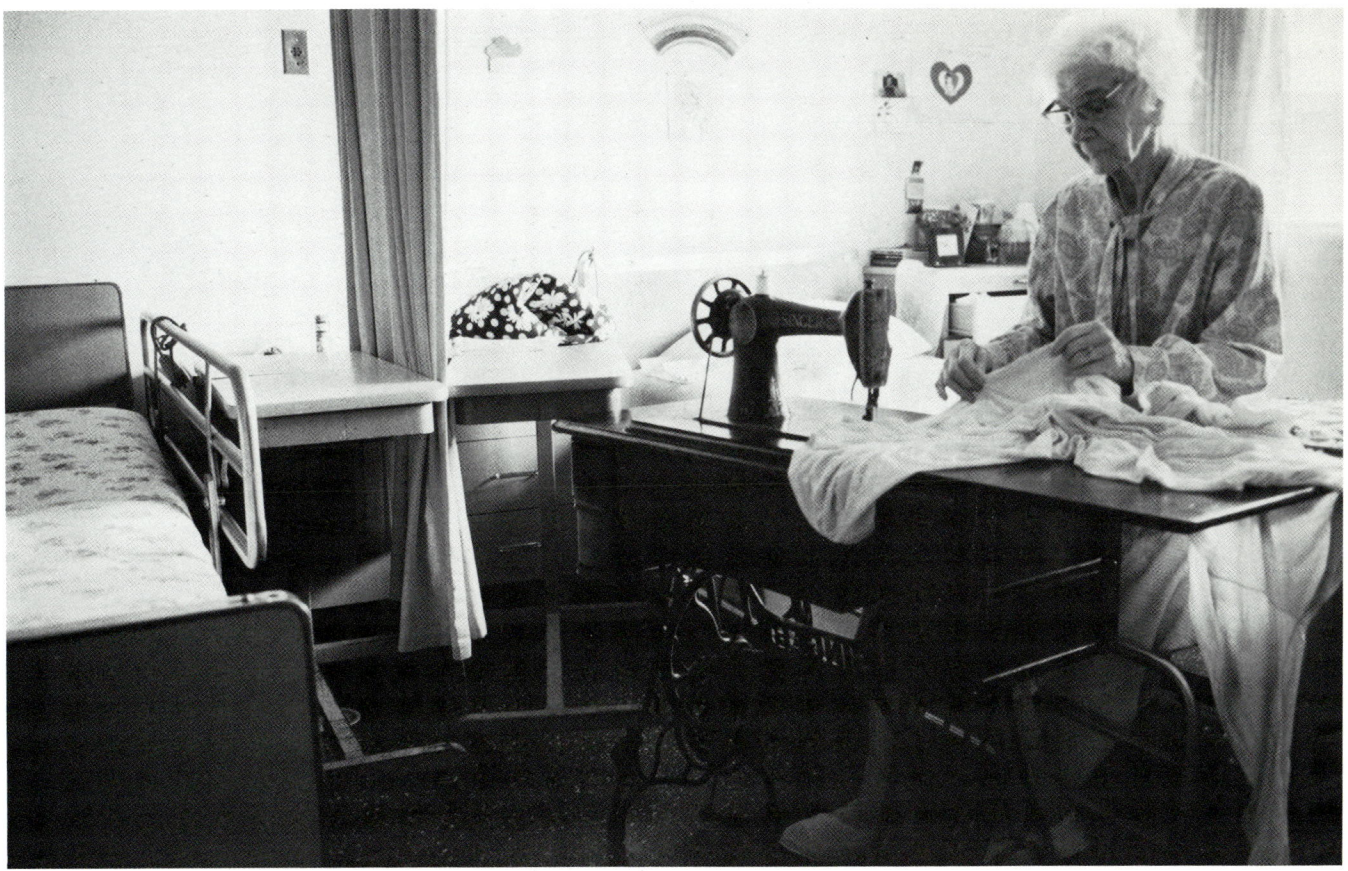

I've had Baby for a long time. When I first got married my husband came home one day and surprised me with Baby. Back then I used to sew all the time and made all of my dresses. Some of them I still wear today.

I haven't used Baby for so long. Opened her up the other day and she's nice as she can be. A little scratched, but a little oil and she will be just fine. She still purrs like a kitten. Look how nice the seams and stitches are. I tell you, Baby is just as good as she has ever been. She's such a grand little baby. Just perfect.

—Josephine

A BOUQUET OF FLOWERS

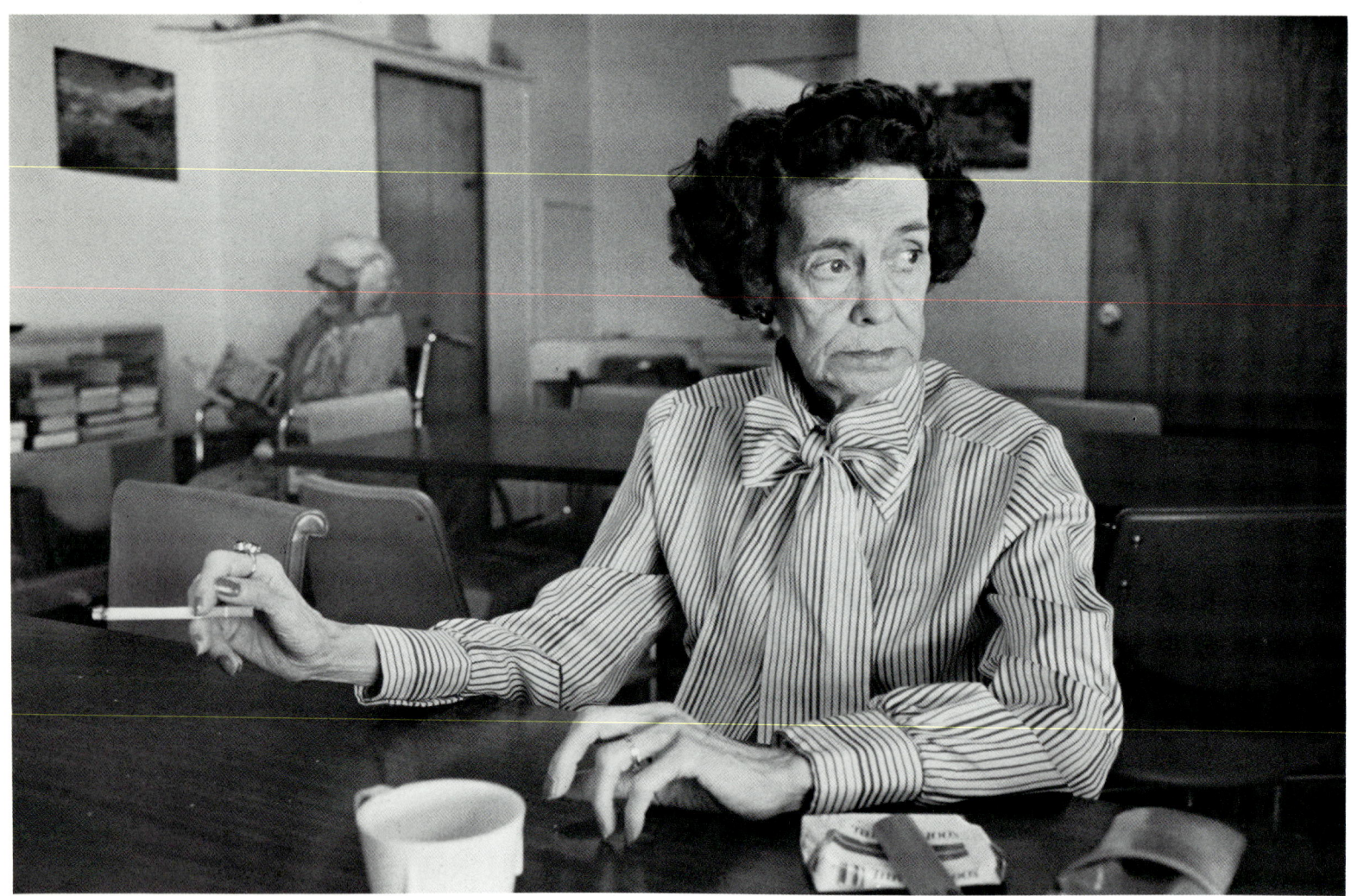

The doctors say I got throat cancer. Now I'm taking radiation and they're going to give me x-ray treatments, chemotherapy, and then they're going to give me a bouquet of flowers for my graveside.

—Bernice

SHE KNEW

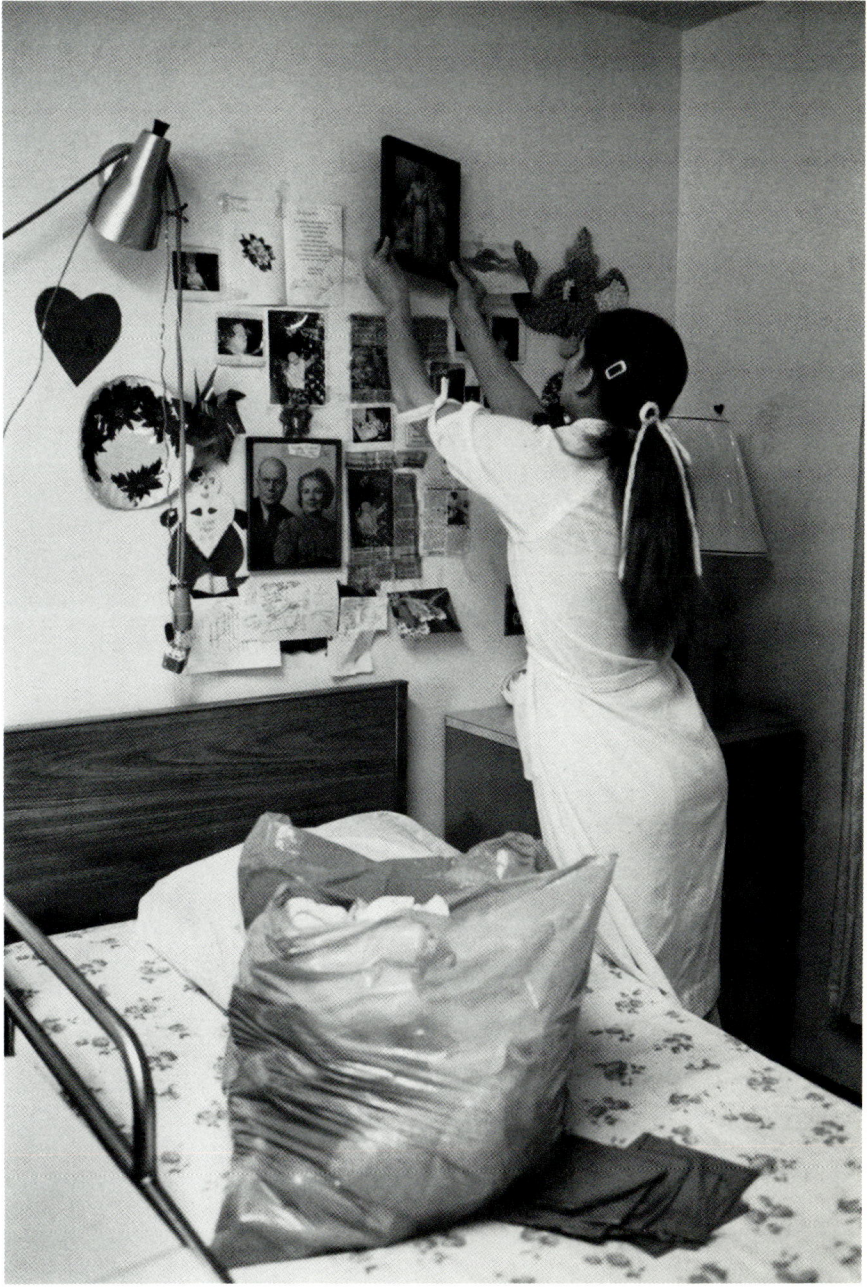

Some of these pictures are old, and I don't know how they're going to travel. Look at the wedding picture—isn't that neat? I would always come in here and look at Cena's pictures. I would say something about them and Cena would say, "Ah, ah, ah," and start waving her hands at me. She knew.

It's sad packing all of her stuff, but it's worse when they die. I'd rather have the biggest mess to clean up than have to pack up someone's stuff after they died. You know they're gone, and you can't do anything about bringing them back.

—Nina

FIFTY FEET

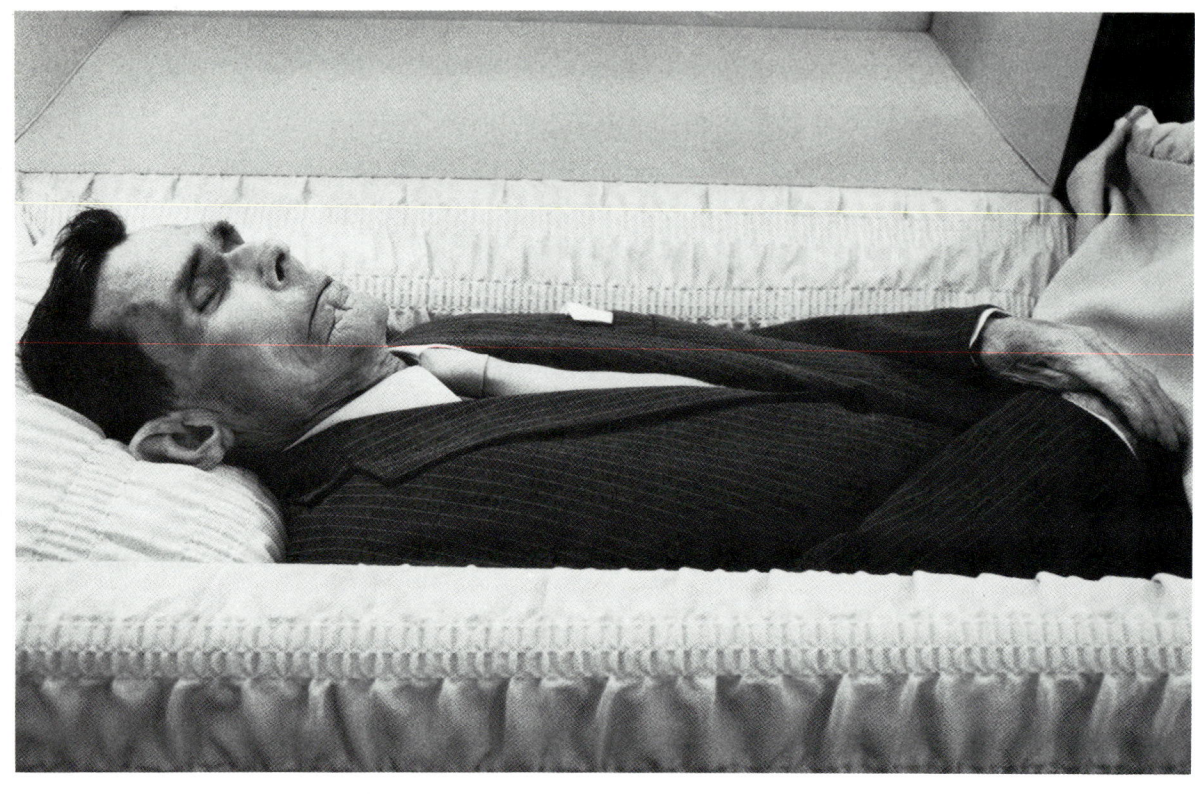

For most of his adult life, Leroy suffered bad health. Despite periodic hospitalizations, however, he was employed full time for many years. He retired in his early fifties, and over the next four years he was in and out of the hospital. During his last hospitalization, his wife died, and he was sent to the nursing home. He lived there for three years before he died. His father Troy, a spry ninety-six, outlived both his sons.

As a kid, Buzz always kept to himself. He was friendly and sociable with people, but he never told anyone about his troubles or his affairs. He didn't talk too much. Buzz was small for his age, but he was awful quick and he could take care of himself. Even his older brother would back off from him, because you didn't know what Buzz would do. He fought to win, not giving a damn what it took. I'll never forget the dive he made when he was nine years old. Just as I looked up, Buzz was going to dive off a cliff. Afraid to holler, I just stood there, but he made a perfect dive. Fifty feet!

I never caught Buzz without any money, he always had money in his pocket. You could give him a pocketknife that wasn't worth a dime and before you knew it, he would have a damned good knife and a little money in his pocket. Just had a knack for horse trading. Never caught Buzz broke. I had him hit me up for money when he had as high as forty-nine dollars in his wallet.

When Buzz was in the Army he got sick and it affected him for the rest of his life. The Army had him in the hospital for over a year. He'd gotten sunstroked in California, and he told me that he nearly went crazy. Then they shipped him to Texas. In a training accident a piece of shrapnel hit him in the foot, knocking a big toe off and part of his foot. After he got out of the Army, every year he'd go to the hospital where they would cut off a little bit more of his foot. I tried to convince the doctors to cut above his ankle so they could put a leg on him. They couldn't 'cause the disease was in his bone. They just cut off a little more each year.

—Troy

VERGIE

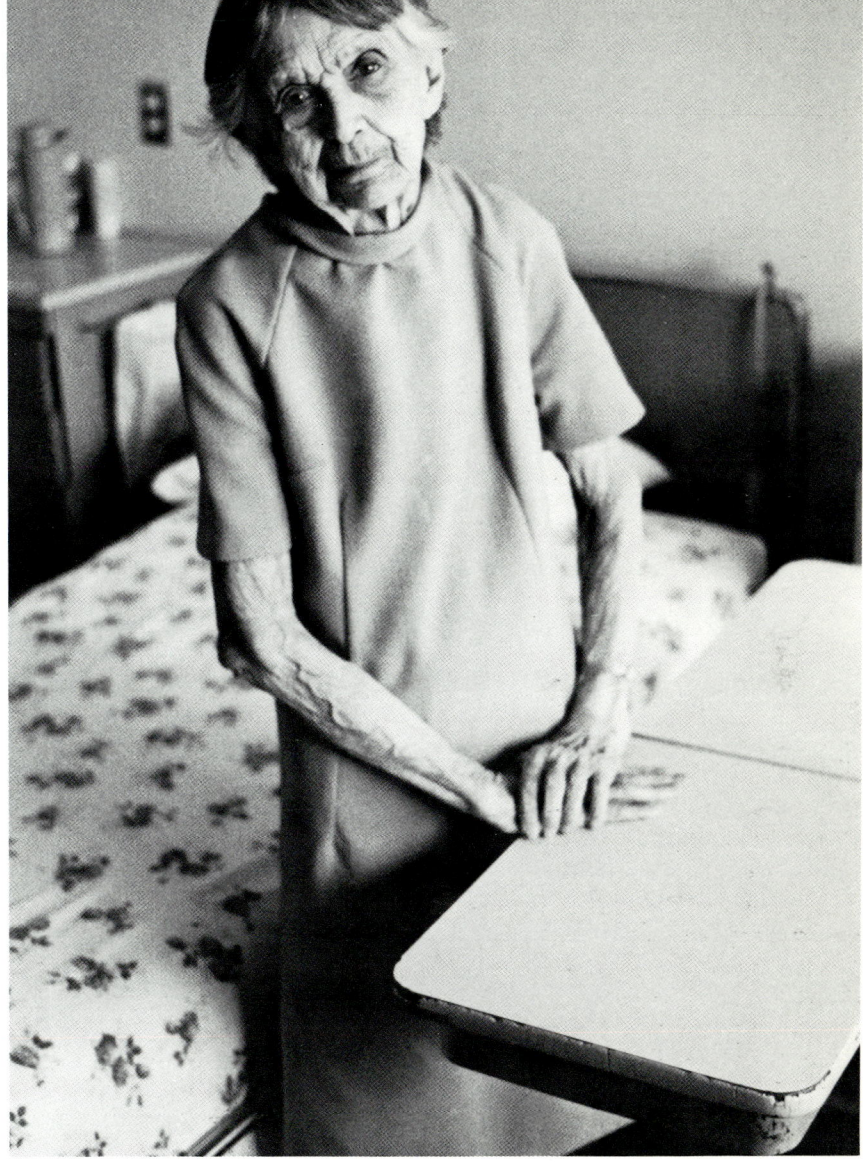

Vergie, a delicate woman in her nineties, rarely left her room. Although she had few possessions to personalize her surroundings, she was particular about the appearance of her room. She helped the aides make her bed in the morning, was meticulous in smoothing out all the wrinkles in her bedspread, and dusted her tabletops. Her clothes were always neatly folded.

This portrait of Vergie was taken two weeks before she died.

VI. The Chill

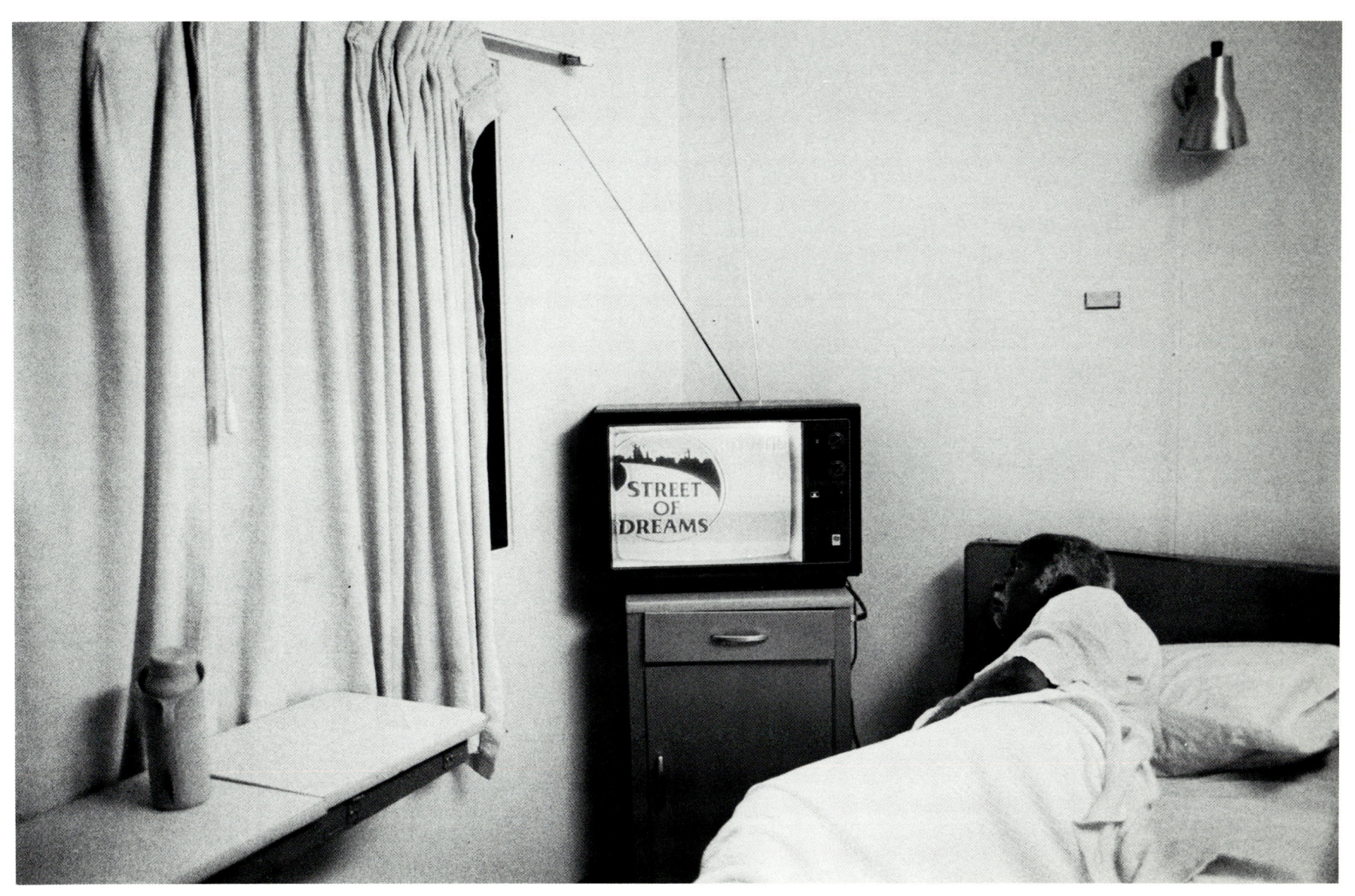

I'VE BEEN FEELING JUST FINE

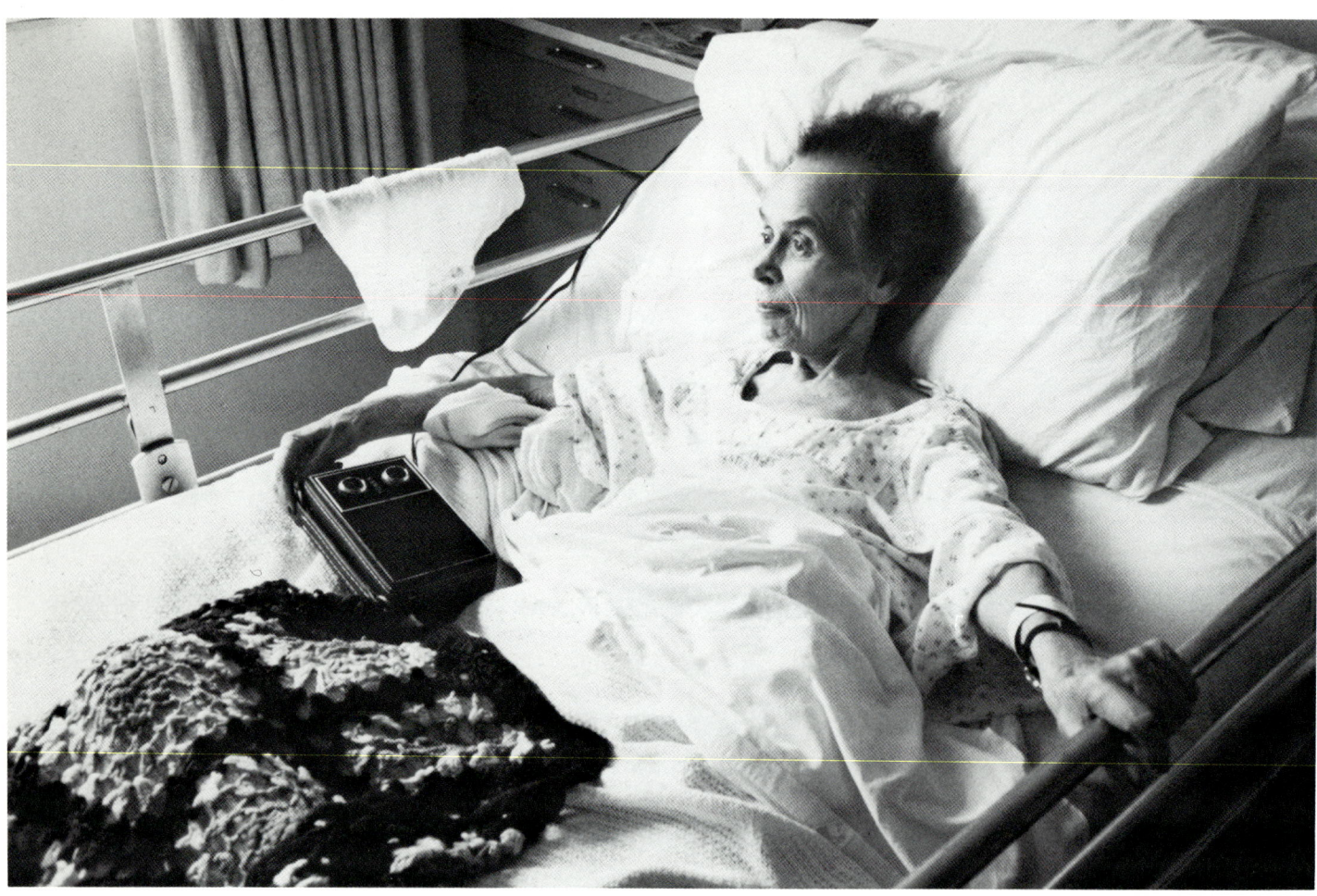

Myrtle is a long-time resident and is known for her cheerful disposition. She never runs out of compliments to the staff and residents about the nursing home. On Town Hall's documentary, "The Hell of Growing Old," she told the audience that "Hundreds of thousands of people just don't know exactly what the rest homes are like. It's a really nice place here. We all get old, and it's a wonderful place to get old." Among other residents, however, she talks about her plans for moving out when she's stronger.

They won't let me out of here until I find a place where someone will look after me. I'm planning to run an ad in the paper for a good, reliable man to look after me. I get three hundred dollars a month, and if he doesn't have any money I'll keep him for a while. But for now I'd settle for one to come in here and talk to me once in a while.

I had a broken hip and on top of that I allowed myself to get anemic. That's what really put me in here. The doctor won't let me out of here until my blood count is way up. Now it's coming along fine, but I've still got to build it up. That's what the doctor said. You need strong blood to build yourself up. But I've been feeling just fine.

—Myrtle

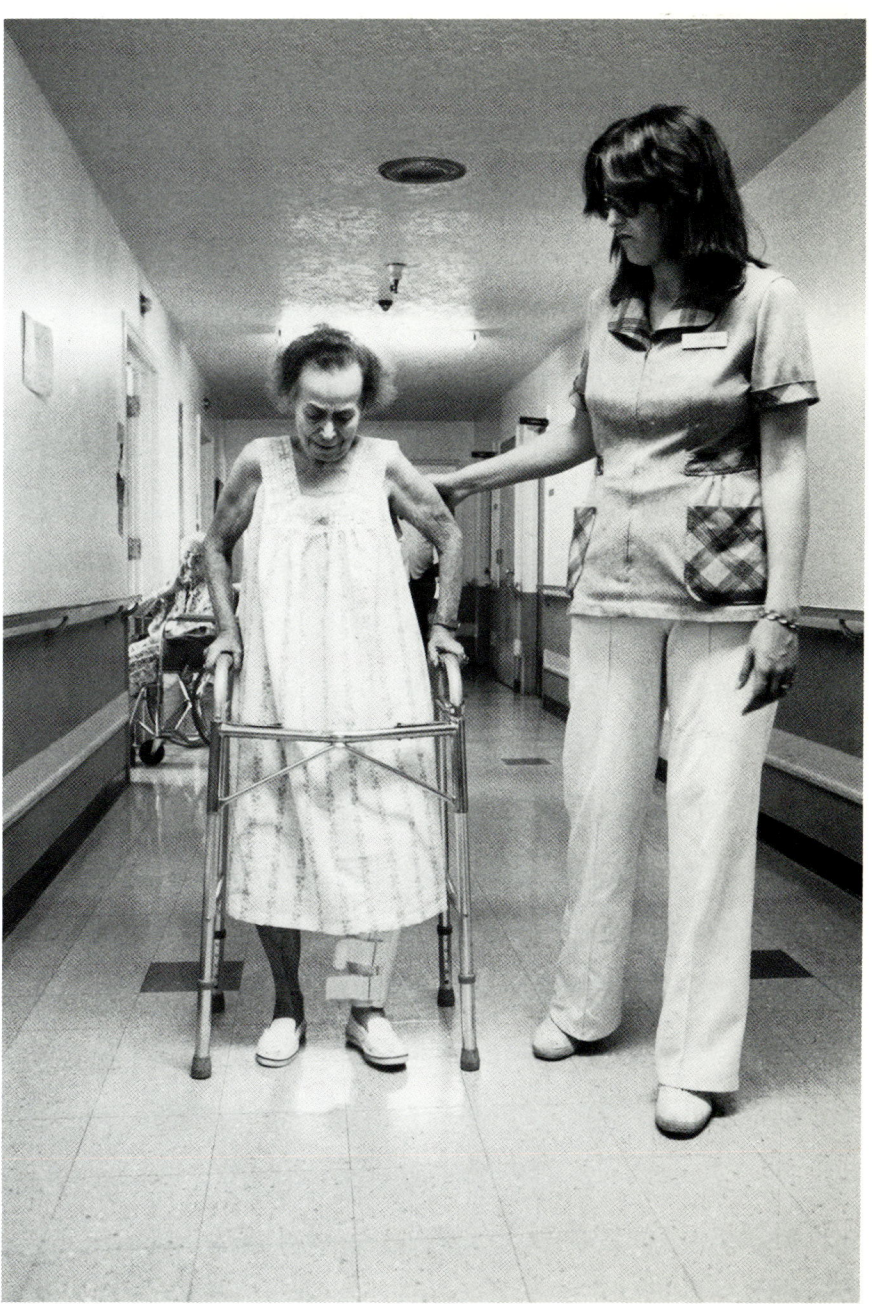

Alma, Myrtle's roommate and friend, is a keen observer of the events shaping Myrtle's life. Always cheerful and very discreet, Alma is a great source of comfort to Myrtle.

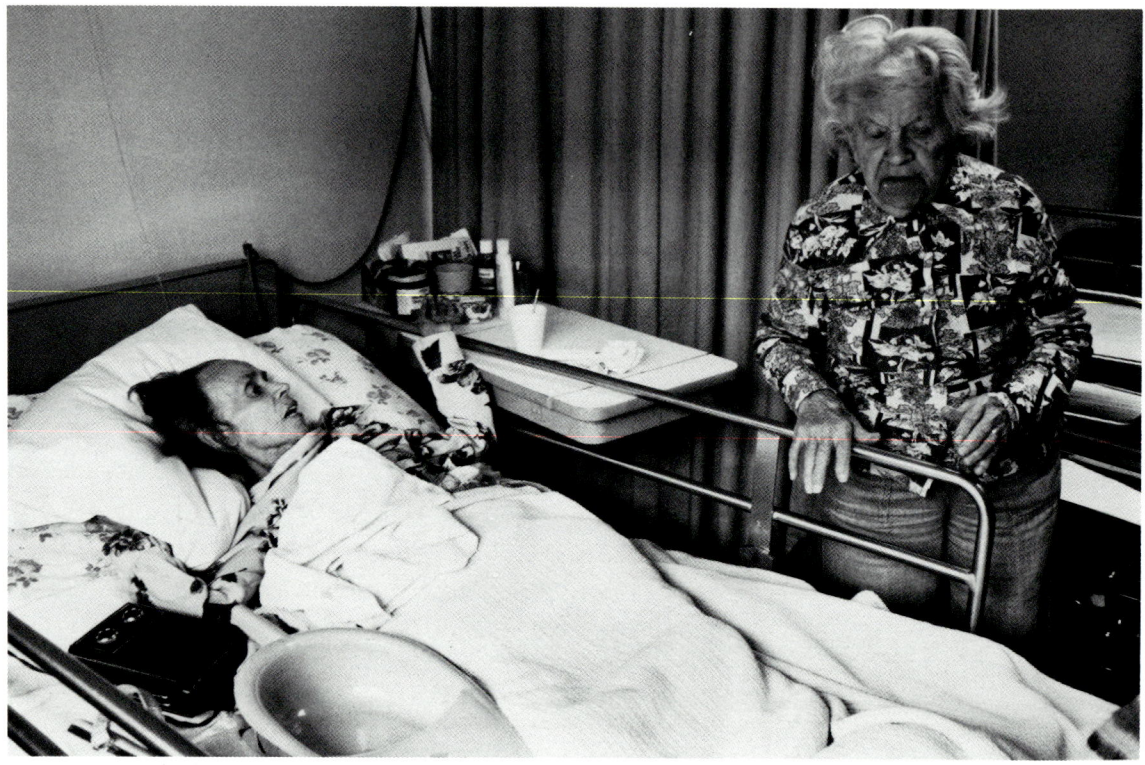

Some of the residents told me that Myrtle has cancer of the blood, but I never mentioned it to her. We didn't talk about it. I don't try to torment people who are sick. The night before she went to the hospital, she dropped the bedpan off the table, makin' an awful racket. I knew she wasn't feeling well. The last couple of days she hadn't eaten and she couldn't even hold fluids. I would try to cheer her up between meals. She would like a cup of tea.

I remember the day she went to the hospital. Before I took my shower, I said goodbye and wished her luck. When I came back, they were dressing her to go to the hospital and the poor dear was crying. I'm going to water her plants until she comes back from the hospital.

—Alma

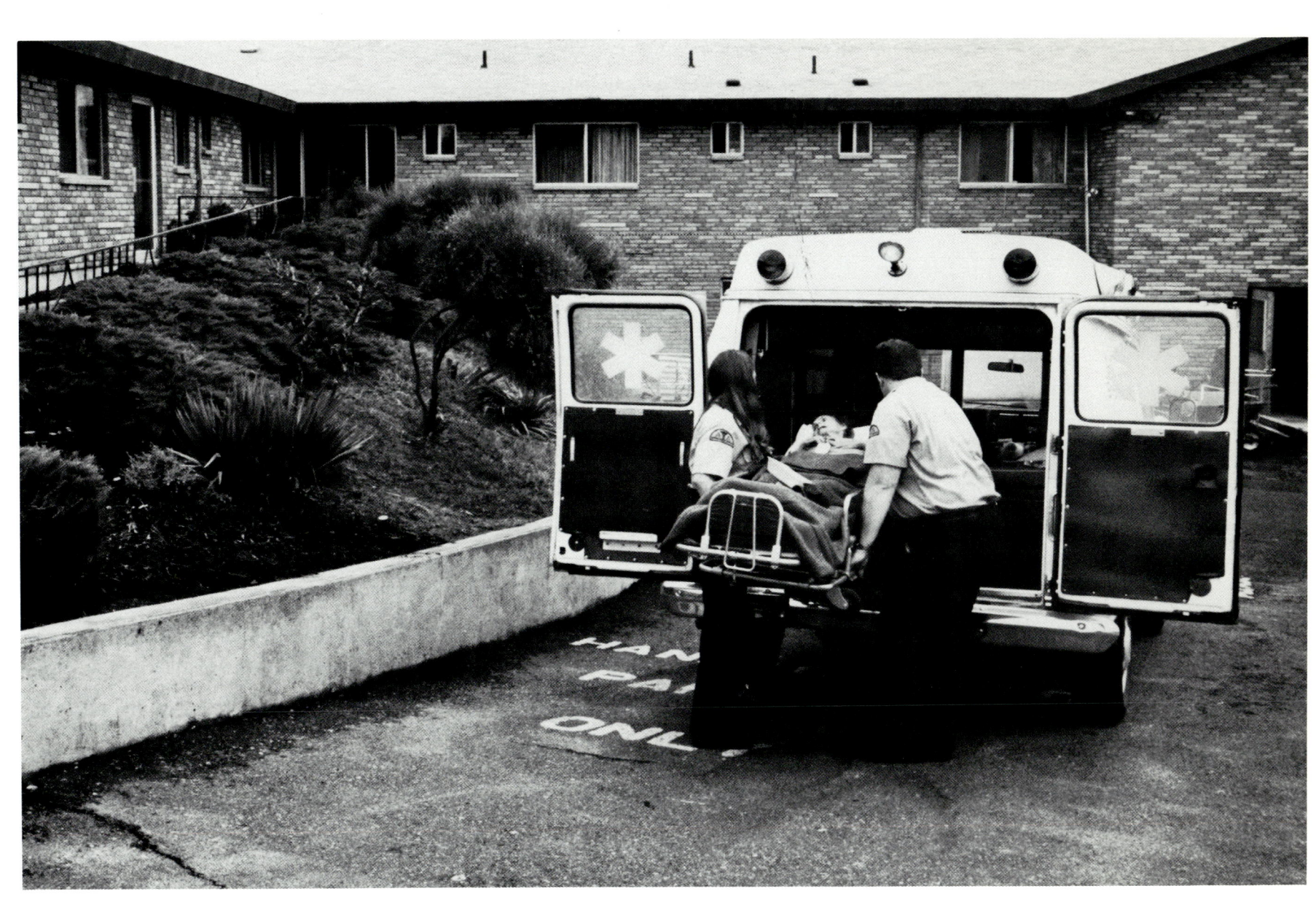

SOMETHING SNAPPED

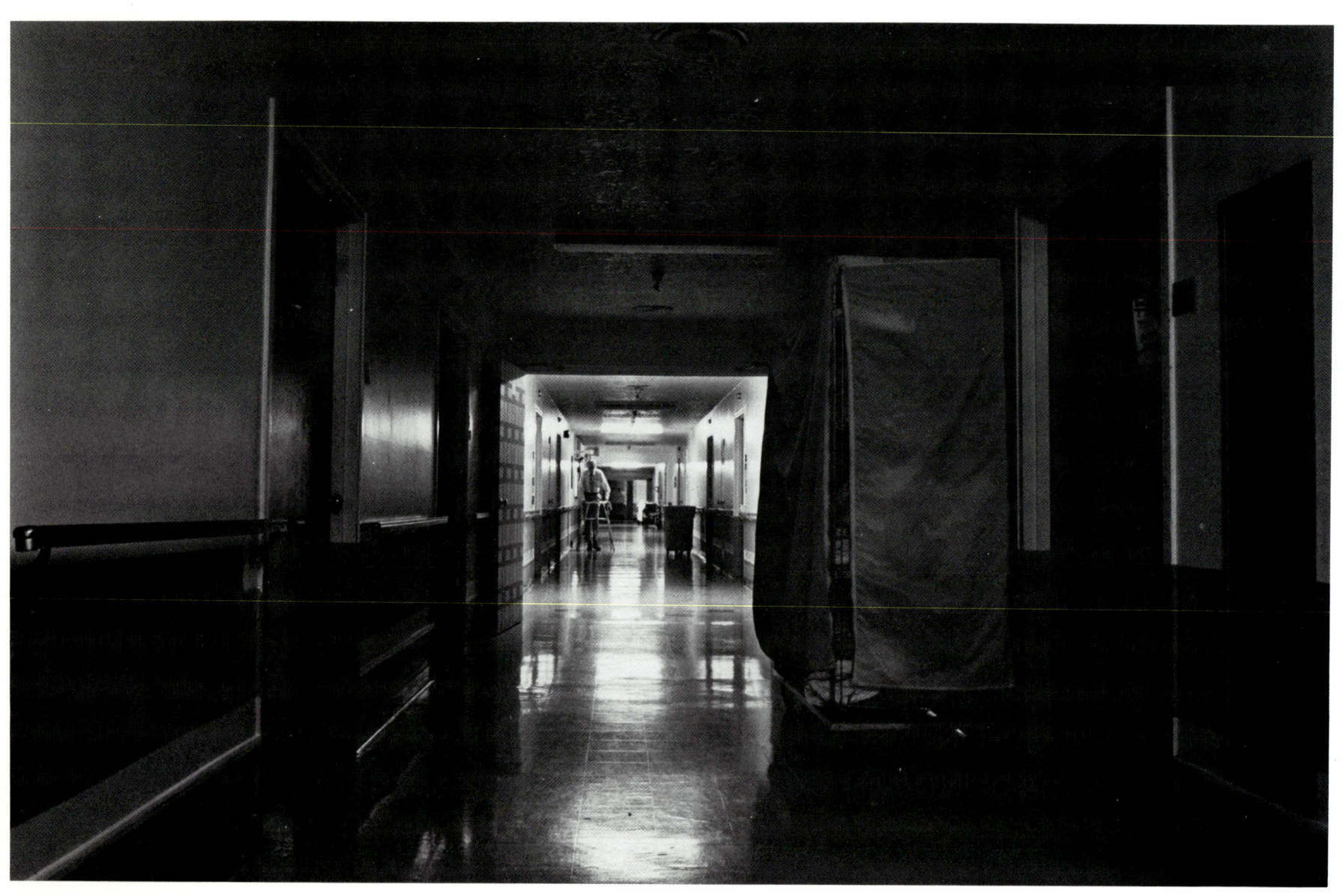

I've got some things I would like to say. I would like to talk about what happened over the weekend. I think that it is important that everyone knows what happened, and what's been done about it, to avoid any rumors or unnecessary fears on your part.

Early Sunday morning one of the aides went rather bananas and hurt at least four people. My best guess is that something snapped. She hit some people, was very rough, scratched some other people. At least four people we know of were involved, and I think there were some other people who didn't report it.

That aide, of course, no longer works here and never will. That kind of behavior is appalling. Neither you people nor anyone else should be treated that way. I know that it is a common fear of people who live in nursing homes that staff can do this kind of stuff to you and get away with it. One of the reasons that I'm here is to let you know that they can't. Anytime that you think that you're being treated roughly, let the nurses know it. If they don't respond, let me know and I will check it out. I'll see that something is done about it. I will not put up with any staff treating you that way.

The facility is also very upset with what happened. This is not behavior expected from the staff. They expect the aides and nurses to treat you with respect and dignity. I think that most of the staff are good people. They really work hard, really try. Something like what happened is something the facility has no way to expect. They really had no control over the fact that it happened. It probably will never happen again. But it could happen again tomorrow. You just don't know.

It's been reported to the police department, and they have been out and investigated it. I've investigated it. Health Division has investigated it. In fact, this thing has been investigated to death. The people who were involved have probably talked to more people in the last few days than they have talked to for months.

I think everyone should be thankful to Donnabelle for her involvement. Donnabelle found out what was happening and kept an eye on the woman, and actually called the police to let them know what was happening. I think the police response was less than adequate. My guess is that the police thought that this woman calling from a nursing home complaining about people is obviously nuts 'cause we all know that people in nursing homes don't make sense.

I think that it would make good sense for everyone in this group to write a letter to the Police Department to tell them what happened: that a resident called to make a complaint and that there was no response. Tell them your feelings about that. I think that they should have come out, at least checked with the nurse to see if there was any problem. I think it's a sign of what people think about nursing homes, and that they don't care to listen to what residents have to say. I'm appalled by that.

—Lonnie, Caseworker

AN OLD BULL'S NECK

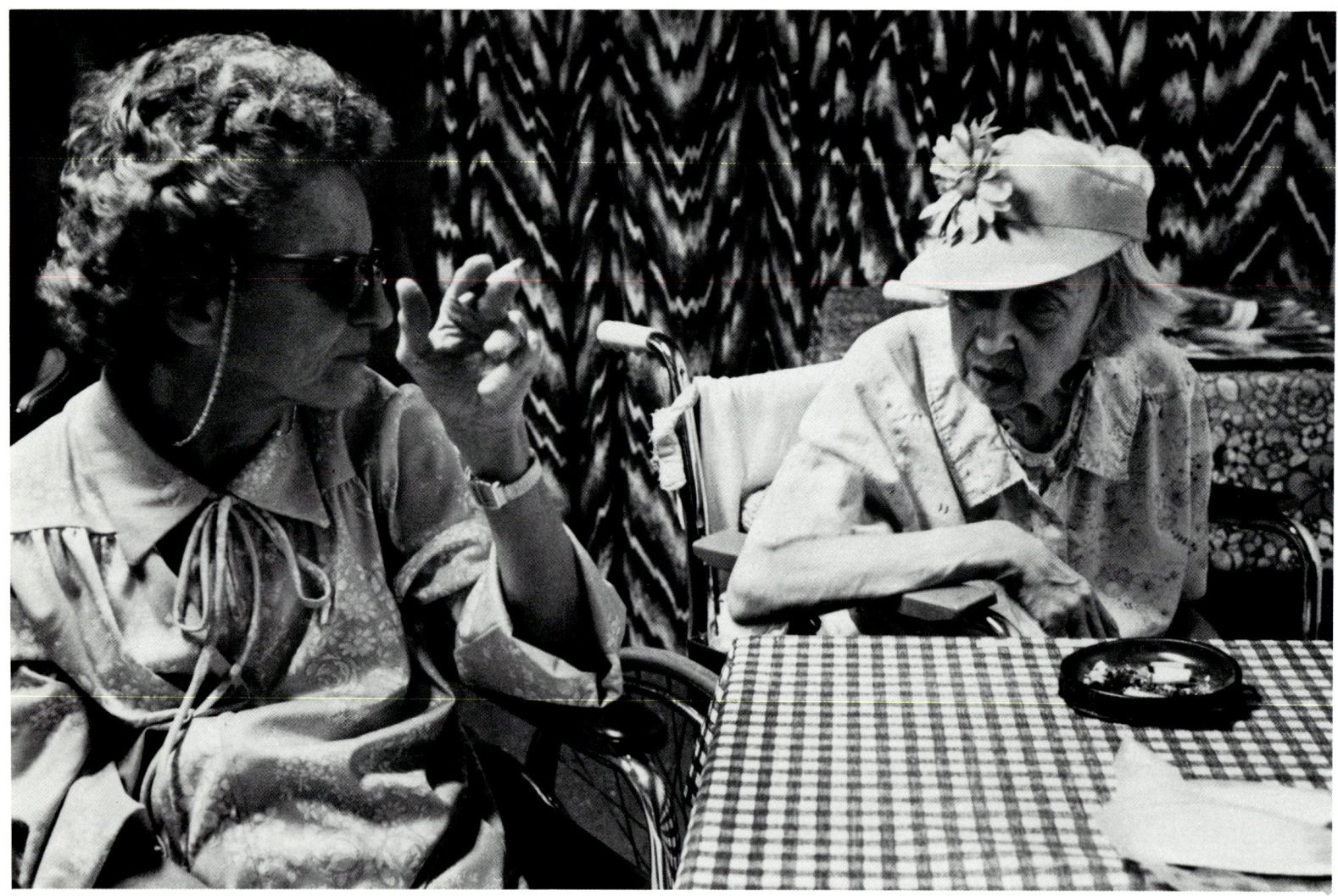

—Hear about that guy who choked to death on a piece of meat?
—Yeah, I heard that the staff tried to turn him every which way but loose and still couldn't get it out of him.
—That meat was so tough, it must have come off an old bull's neck.

THEY DO IT TO OLD PEOPLE

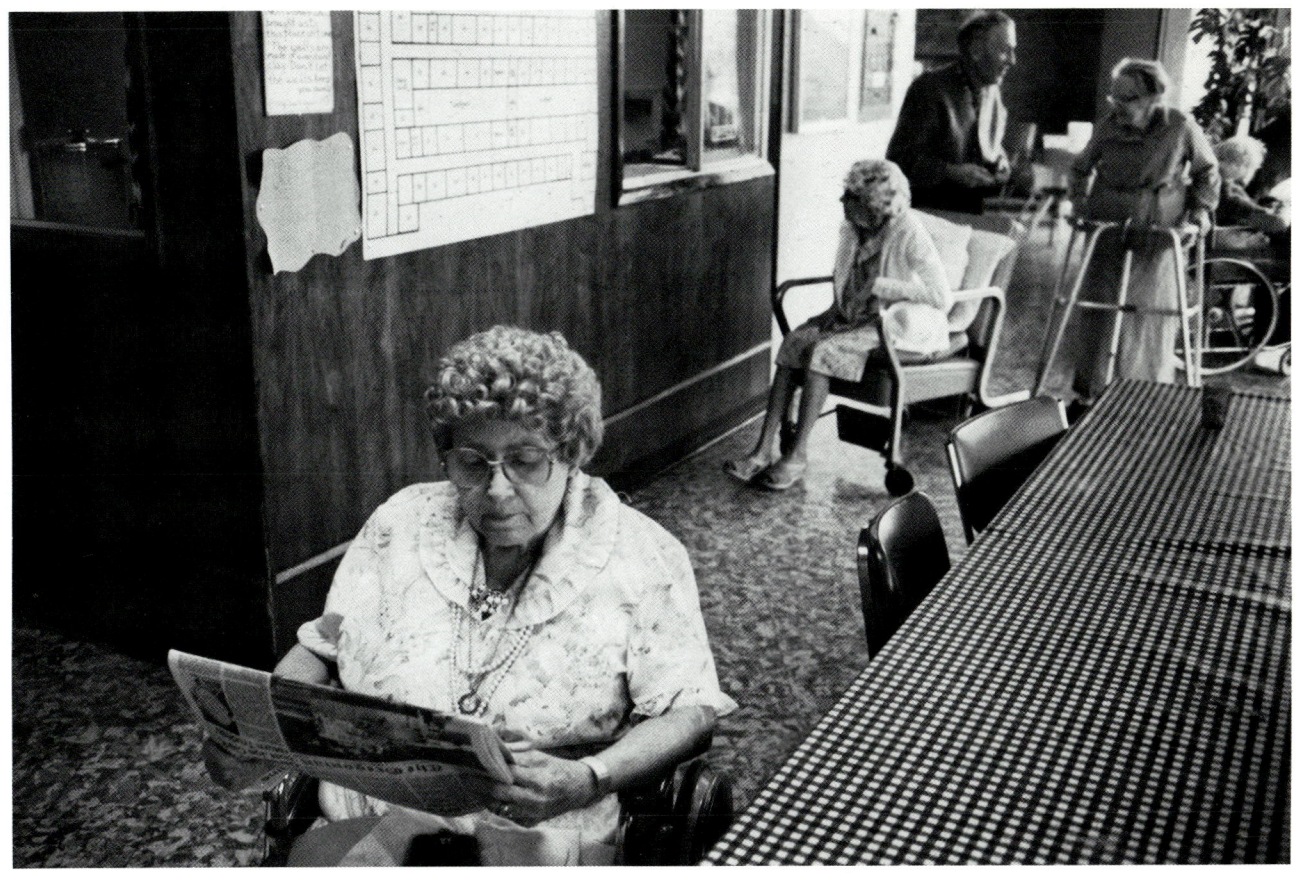

You wonder what's going on in the world. You're glad that you're not out there, I guess. You feel kind of safe in here. I wouldn't want to go out on the street by myself. Some of those kids might come along and tip your wheelchair over. They do it to old people. You read about it all the time in the newspaper. Just yesterday somebody tried to break into my sister's house. Somebody saw him and called the police. He was only a kid. Seventeen years old! If the police hadn't come and got him, he might have killed her. You read about violence all the time in the paper. It's sickening.

—Georgia

I DON'T WANT TO DIE

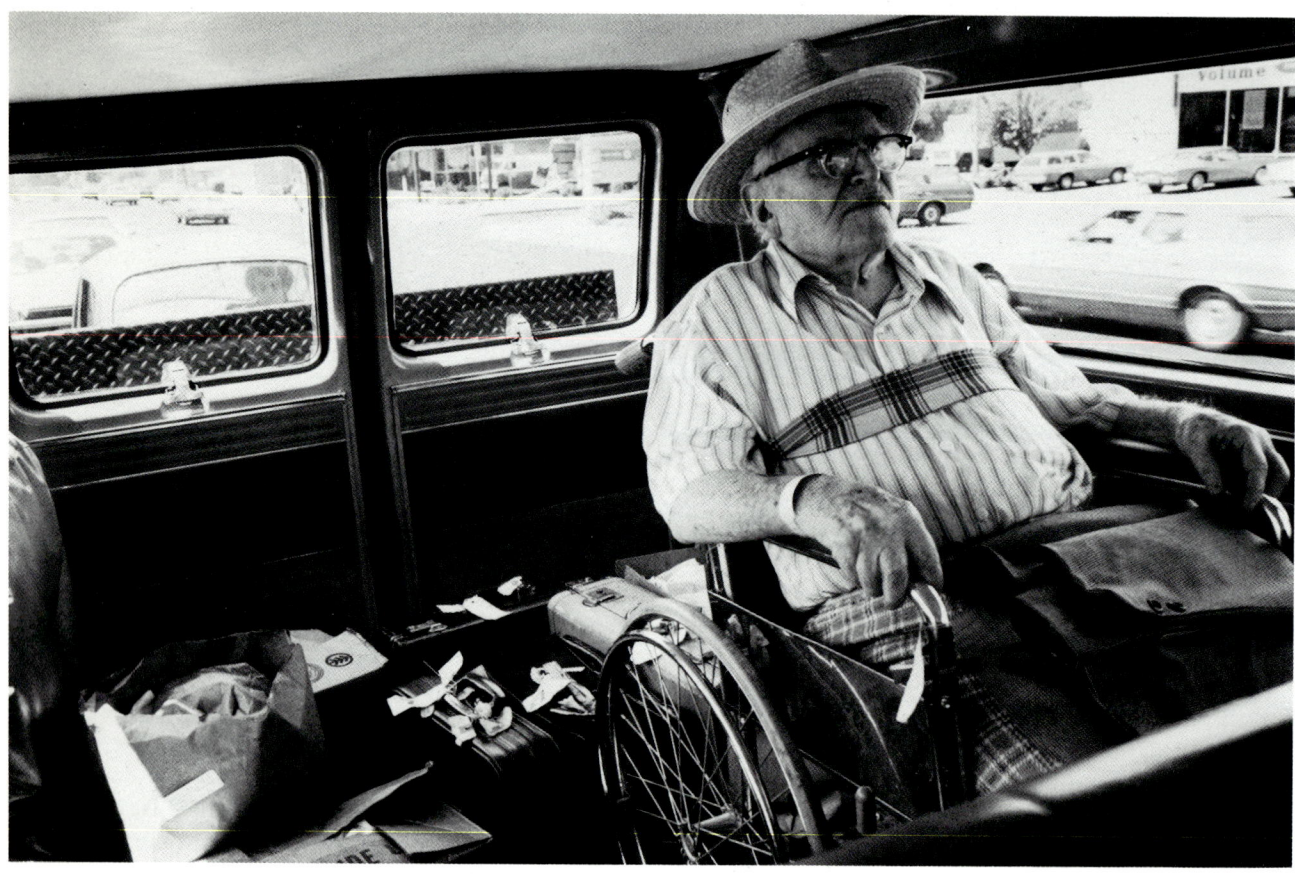

Louis is a former traveling salesman from the Midwest. In his travels, he frequently opened new accounts at the local banks, so that he would never be caught short. For unknown reasons, he relocated to the Northwest later in his life, where he continued his nomadic life style on a smaller scale—moving from one hotel to another.

Despite his declining health and increasing difficulty in managing his personal affairs, Louis insists on doing things his own way. His abrasive personality combined with his secretiveness about his personal affairs hasn't endeared him to most people. Yet he has a few admirers. A maid, Ruby, who knows Louis from his previous stays at the Heathman Hotel, a facility that once catered to elderly pensioners and former mental patients, considers Louis a bona fide character. "Certainly doesn't take any crap off nobody. He kind of reminds me of a little bantam rooster, always ready to mix it up. You know, banties are noted for being fighters."

Rob and I first got to know Louis in the week before he was transferred to the nursing home from the VA Hospital where he had been convalescing from an illness. Louis said the social worker who had picked out the home told him that it is a very nice place and the people are very friendly. "I'll have to take his word for it. That's what I'm looking for—to meet friendly people. I make friends easily, but I also make enemies."

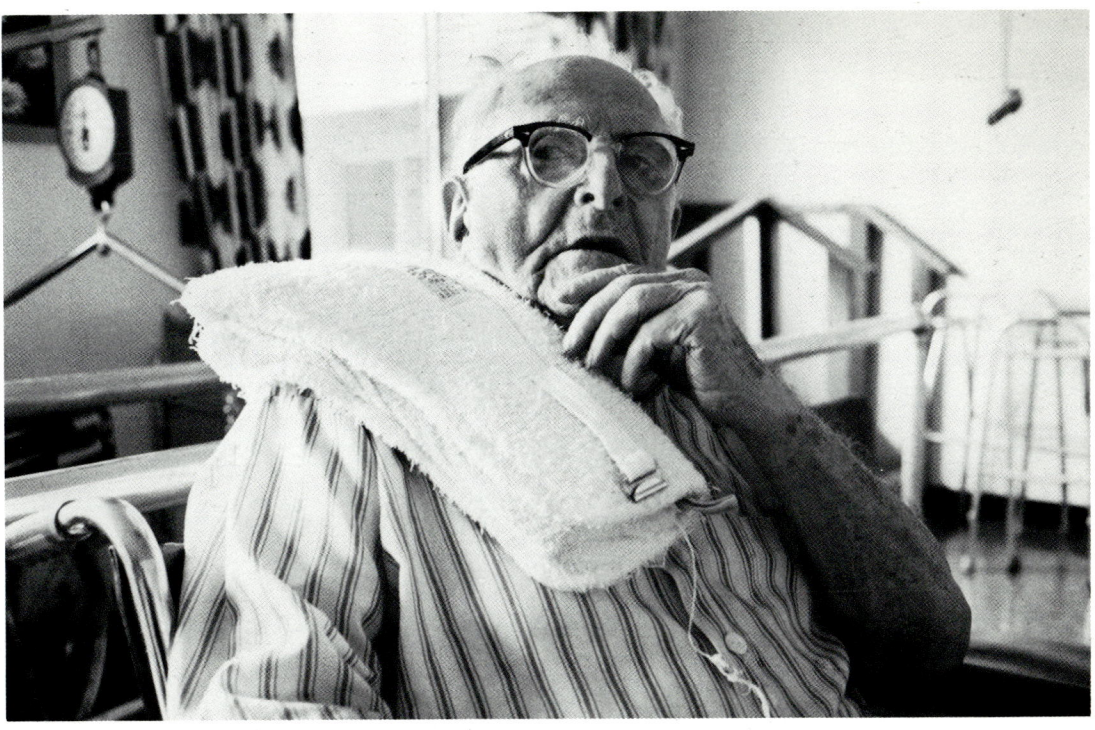

I've been in a lot of different nursing homes, and I'll tell you, the private homes are in it merely for the money. I lived in a private nursing home downstate, for two-and-a-half years, and they robbed me of my life savings—eleven thousand dollars. Just figure it out—how many years I had to work to save that up. And not only that, the place was crooked. They made mistakes and charged me for them. One time they charged me four hundred dollars for a mistake they made. On top of that, the doctor charged me a full forty dollars whenever he examined me. And then the medication. I figured it up—over eleven thousand dollars.

After the nursing home, I lived in a motel. They charged me sixty dollars a week for a TV and telephone. Then I moved to a cheaper place, a motel where I paid fifty-two dollars a week. The only thing I got there was a TV, a bed to sleep on, and myself. Eventually a friend of mine got me a place at a retirement home for four hundred dollars a month. I didn't like that either, so I left.

I took a bus up to Portland and went to a nursing home there. I had negotiated with them beforehand to pay twenty dollars a day. It wasn't a bad place, even though there were mostly women there. But then they suggested that I give them a two-thousand-dollar donation. I told them I'd have to wait and see how much I liked the place. One of the social workers said, "What's the difference? If you run out of money, you can go on relief." I just can't go for that. I've never been on relief, and I never want to go on relief as long as I live. A couple of weeks later they insisted that I pay, so I left and moved into a hotel. . . .

Wherever I go, everybody wants money. That's all they're interested in. The one good thing about the nursing home I'm in now is that it won't cost me a cent. The VA will pay my bill for the first six months because of my recent illness. The way the cost of living is today, I couldn't afford to pay it all myself.

I fell down in the bathroom. I slipped in a puddle of piss, breaking my finger and wrenching my shoulder. Eight men use the bathroom and some of them are pretty careless, pissing all over the floor. So I complained to the administrator. I told him that I was going to sue the nursing home. Well, he told me that it's against the law to put carpeting on the floor. Why the hell is it against the law? The floor is slippery. A lot of people have fallen.

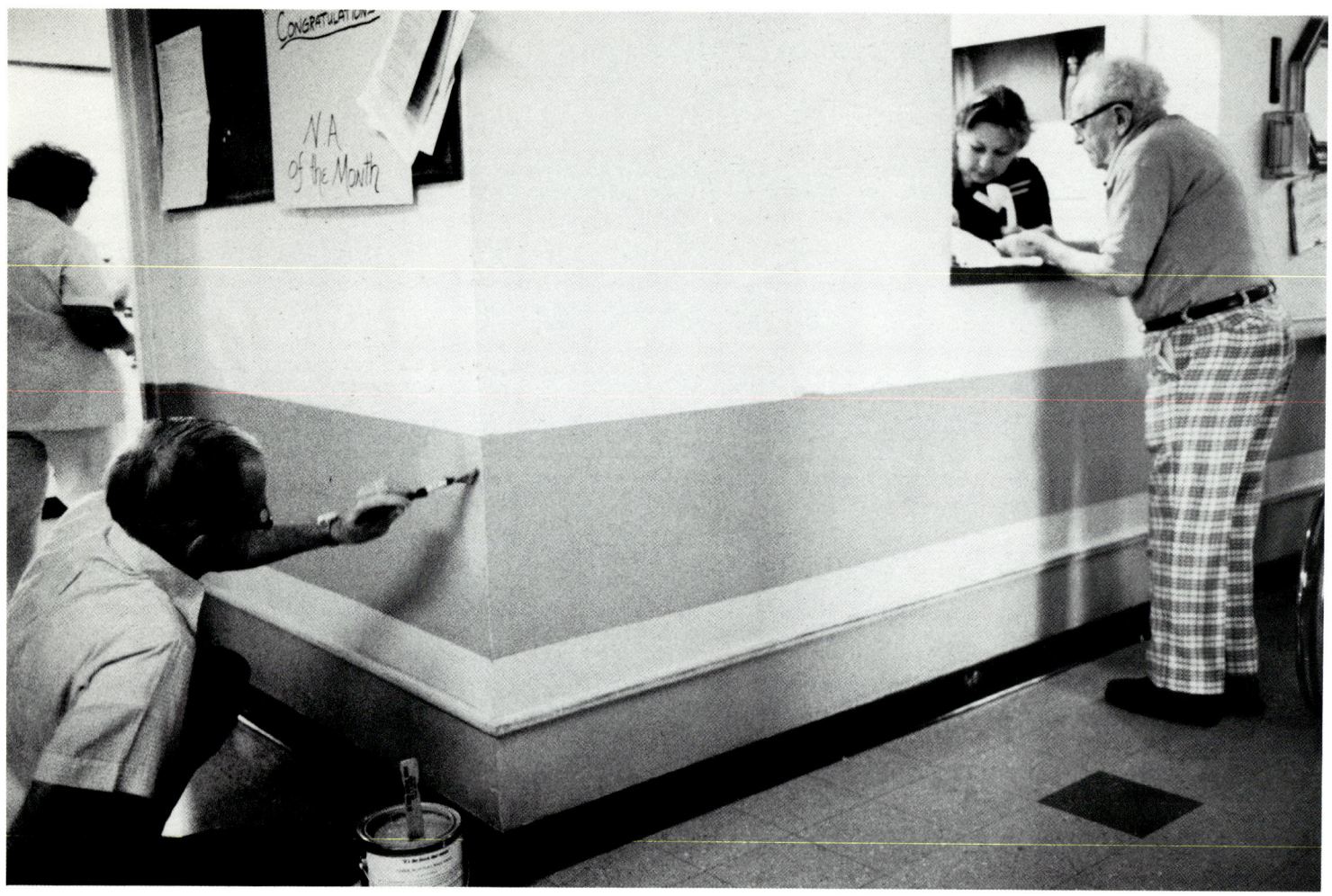

I'm moving out of here. My VA contract expired and the administrator told me I gotta pay a thousand a month to stay here. Well I told the son of a bitch to go to hell. A thousand dollars a month—that's highway robbery. I'm going to call the Heathman Hotel and get a room. I lived there before I went to the VA Hospital. I can live cheap there.

I'm eighty-three. I'm one of the boys who made it. I want to live. I don't want to die.

—Louis

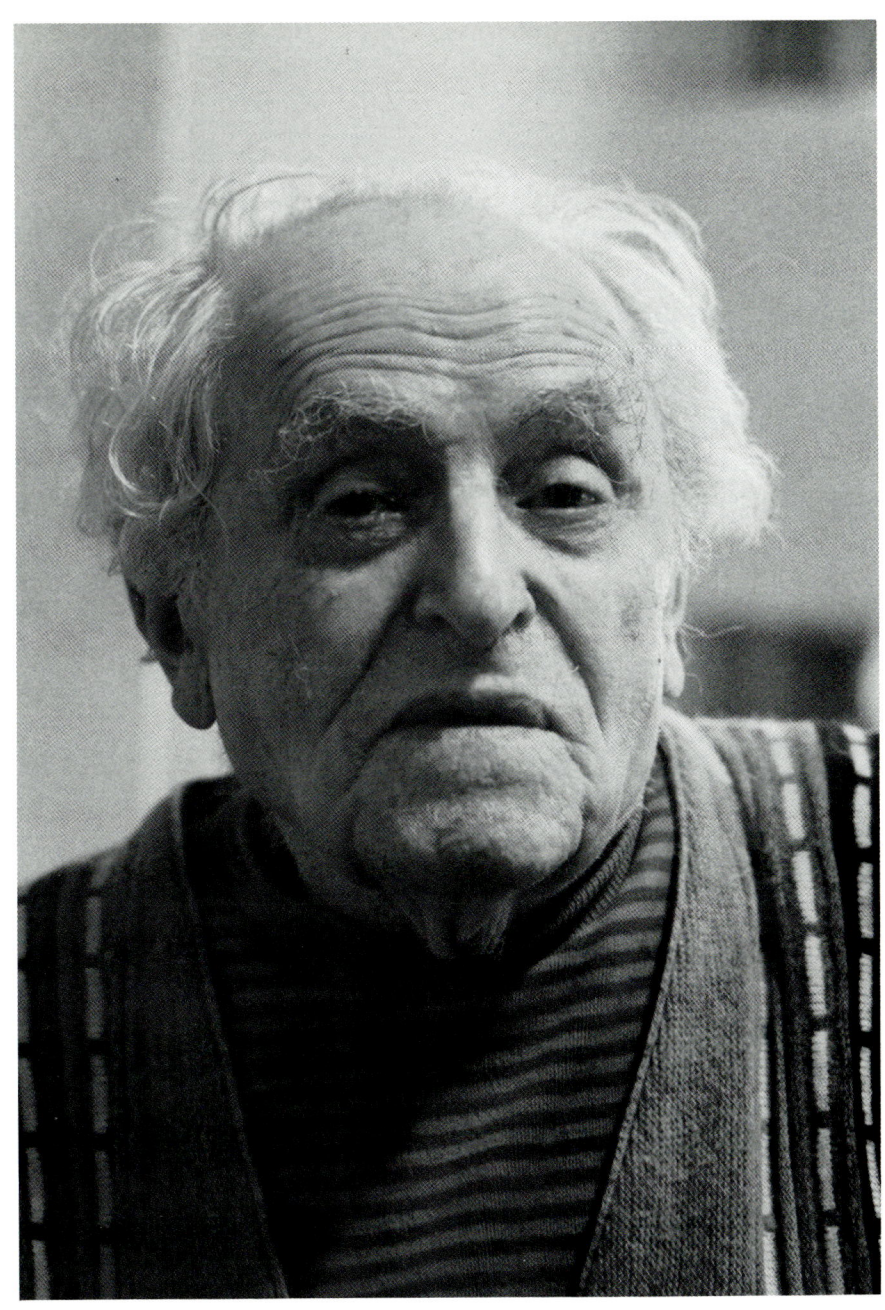

For about a half year Louis seemed reasonably content with his accommodations at the Heathman. He was well known by several of the staff and they respected his need for privacy. Louis was mostly content to stay in his room, where he would rummage through his boxes of personal records, occasionally leaving to play cribbage with several of the residents or to go to a nearby barber college for a haircut. Yet he talked incessantly about moving downstate. We offered to drive Louis, but every time we would show up early in the morning to take him, he had some excuse—he didn't feel well or he needed several more weeks to tie up loose ends. Then, unexpectedly, the Heathman was condemned by the city (later to be refurbished into a luxury hotel bearing the same name). Louis and the other residents were forced to move.

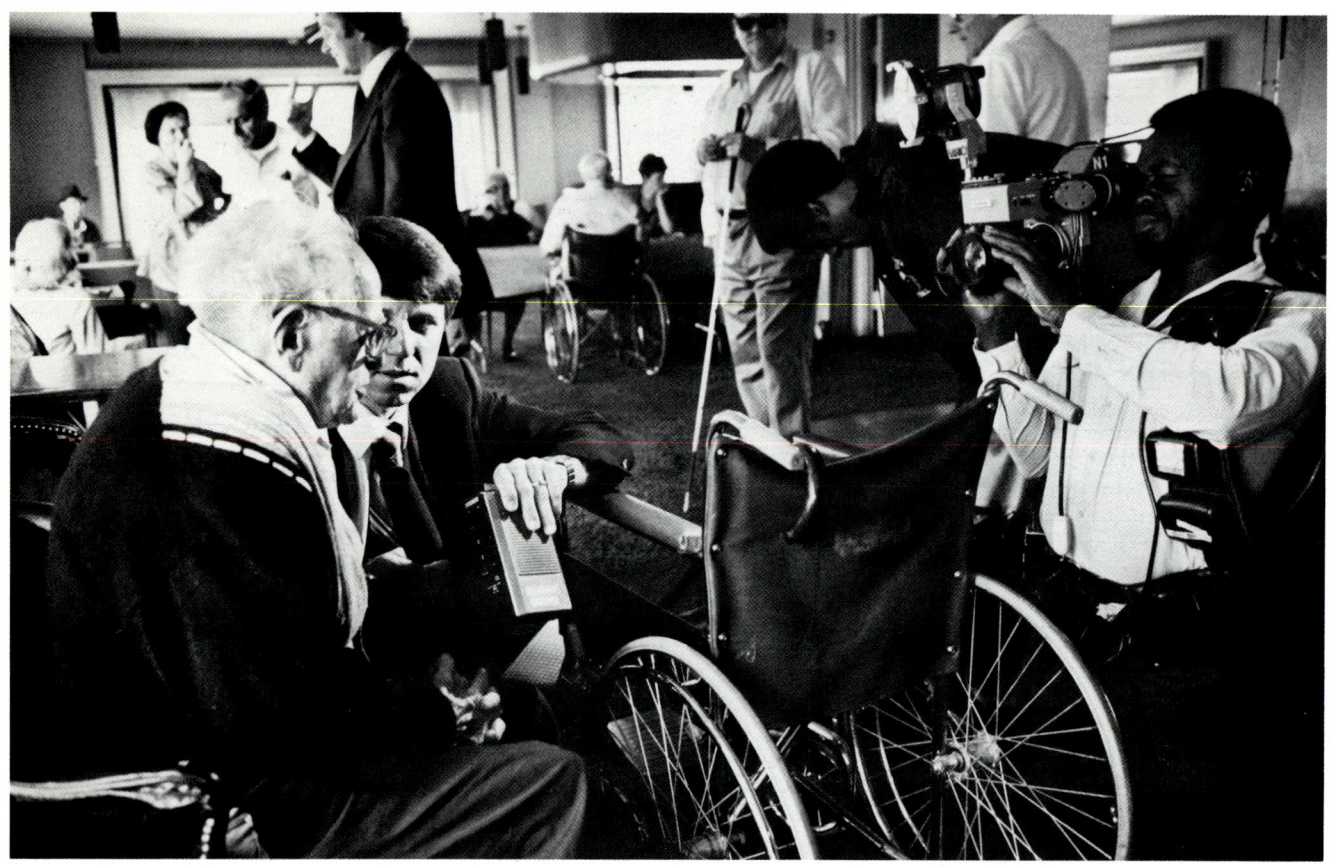

I don't know what's happening. They tell me we have to move out of the hotel Monday. The place is crawling with TV people, all asking the same goddamned questions. How do I feel about getting kicked out of here? Where am I going to live? I'm scared, and I'm too sick to do anything. I can't even walk, can't get around. What can I do? I gotta face the future but I don't know what it looks like.

—Louis

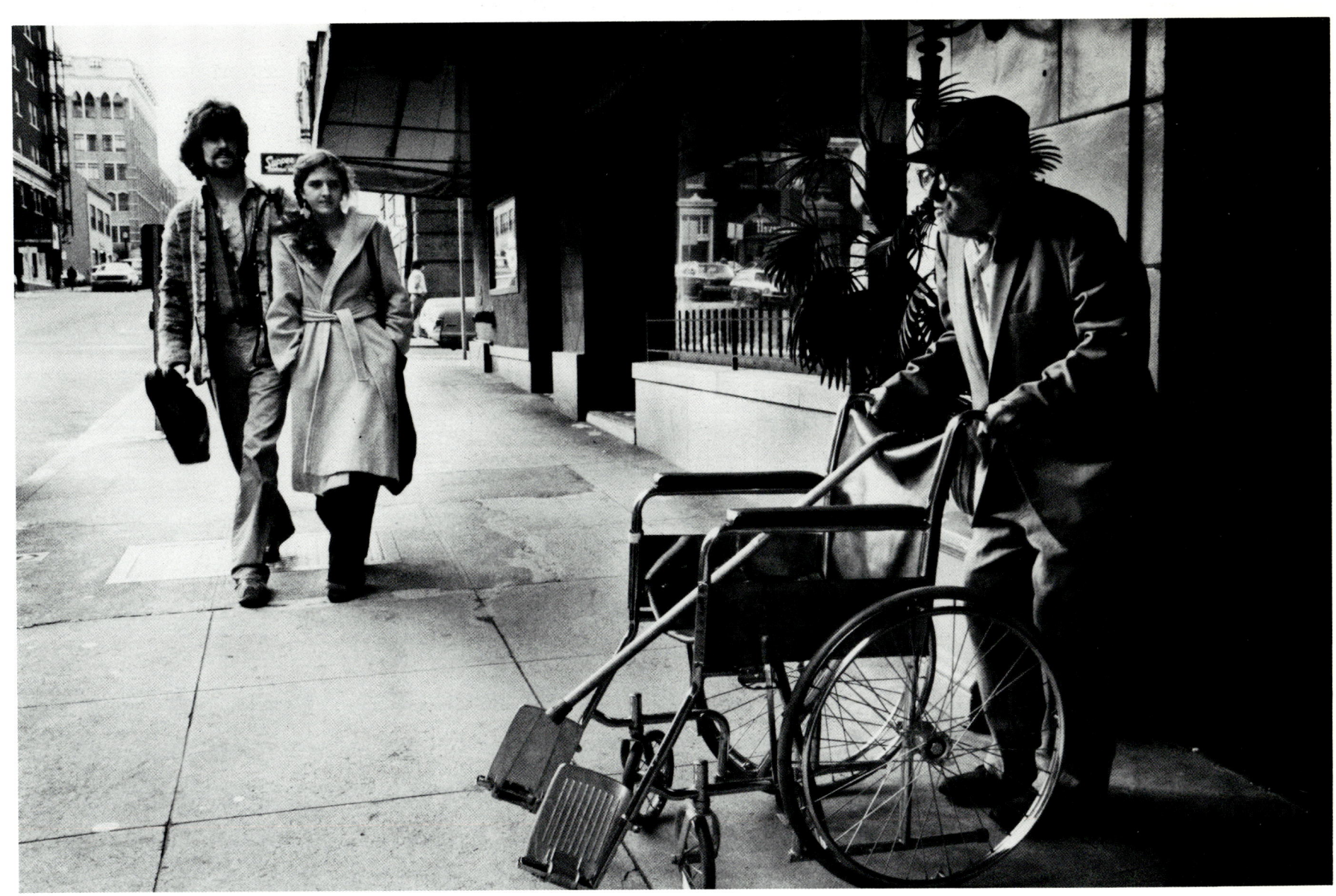

He Died Up In 18

The day before old man Ball died, I took him a letter. He was very alert and he could read it. Then there was Mr. Jones over in Room 57. I didn't wake him up to deliver his mail because he had a cold towel on his head and he looked more dead than alive. I didn't think he would last another day, and he didn't. But I was surprised when old George went. I wasn't sorry, though, because he was a very sick man. He died up in 18. He had been in the hospital and they brought him back. He was awful sick, yelling out for his mother. He must have been very close to her. I went up to the end of the hall and when I came back everything was silent. He was gone.

—Georgia

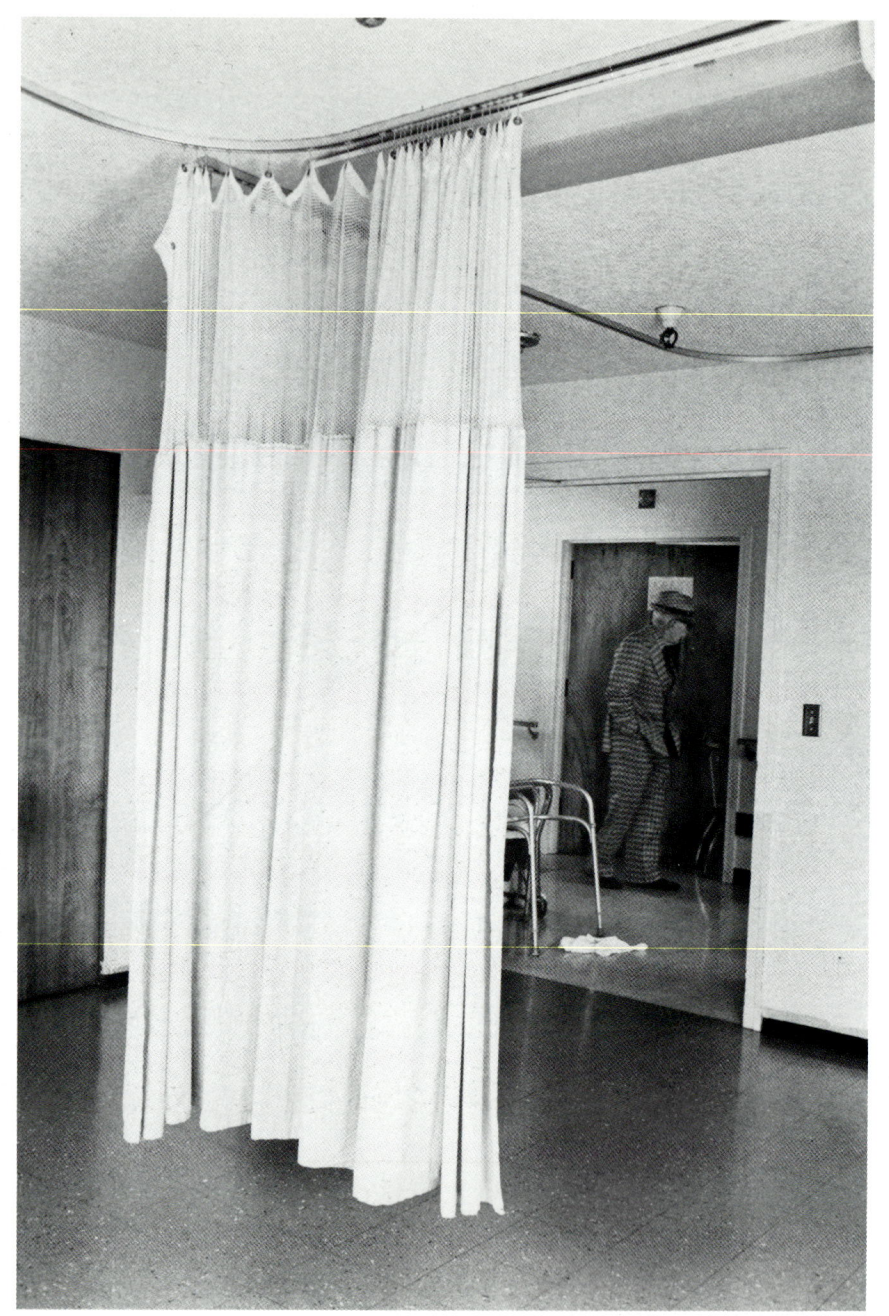

AFTER MIDNIGHT

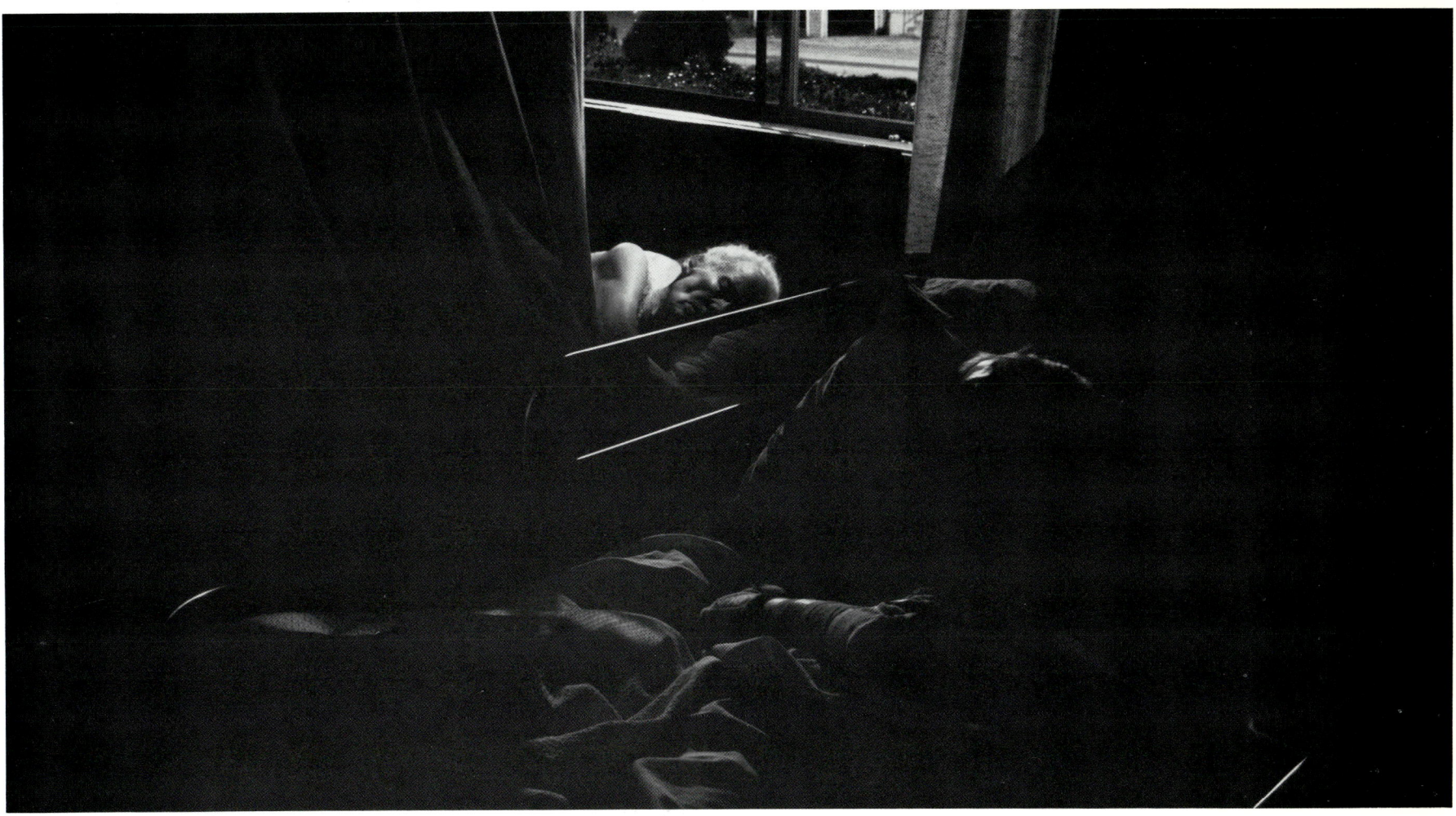

It was after midnight and I was lying in bed. I felt that somebody was in the room—a man with big legs standing on my roommate's bed. He jumped. Just when he was about to land on my chest, I woke up screaming. I guess that makes me kinda nuts.

—Jo

WAITING

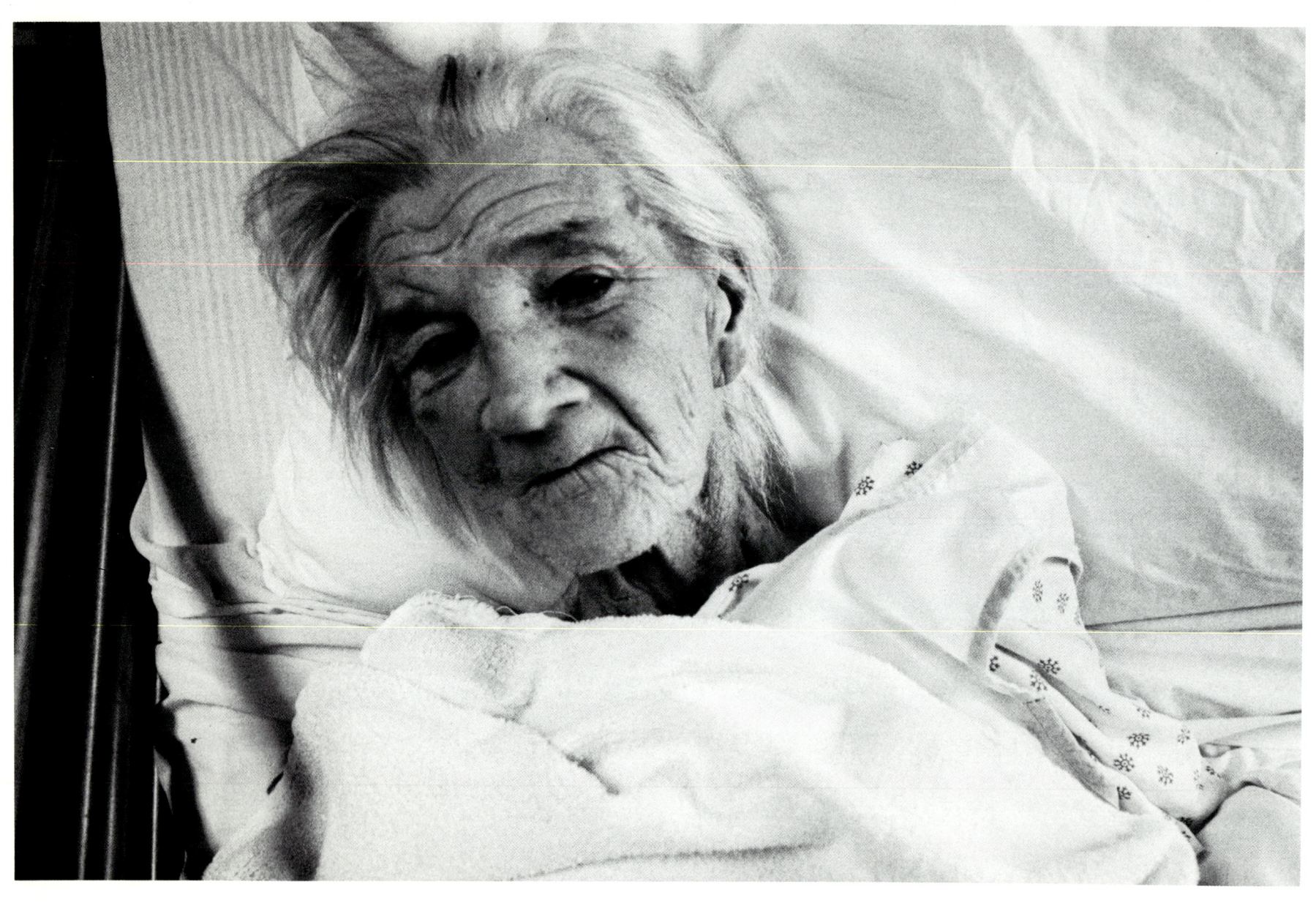

I am so on edge. I can't hardly talk. I'm so ripped up inside that I don't know what to do or say. I've just quit doin' things. I'm gone. I can't pray like I used to. I don't know anything about it, but I've got to go through it. I'm on the way. I don't know what to do. If I could just lie down in the pasture. But I can't. It comes to you so hard, waiting here.

—Josephine

VII. Keeping On, Moving On

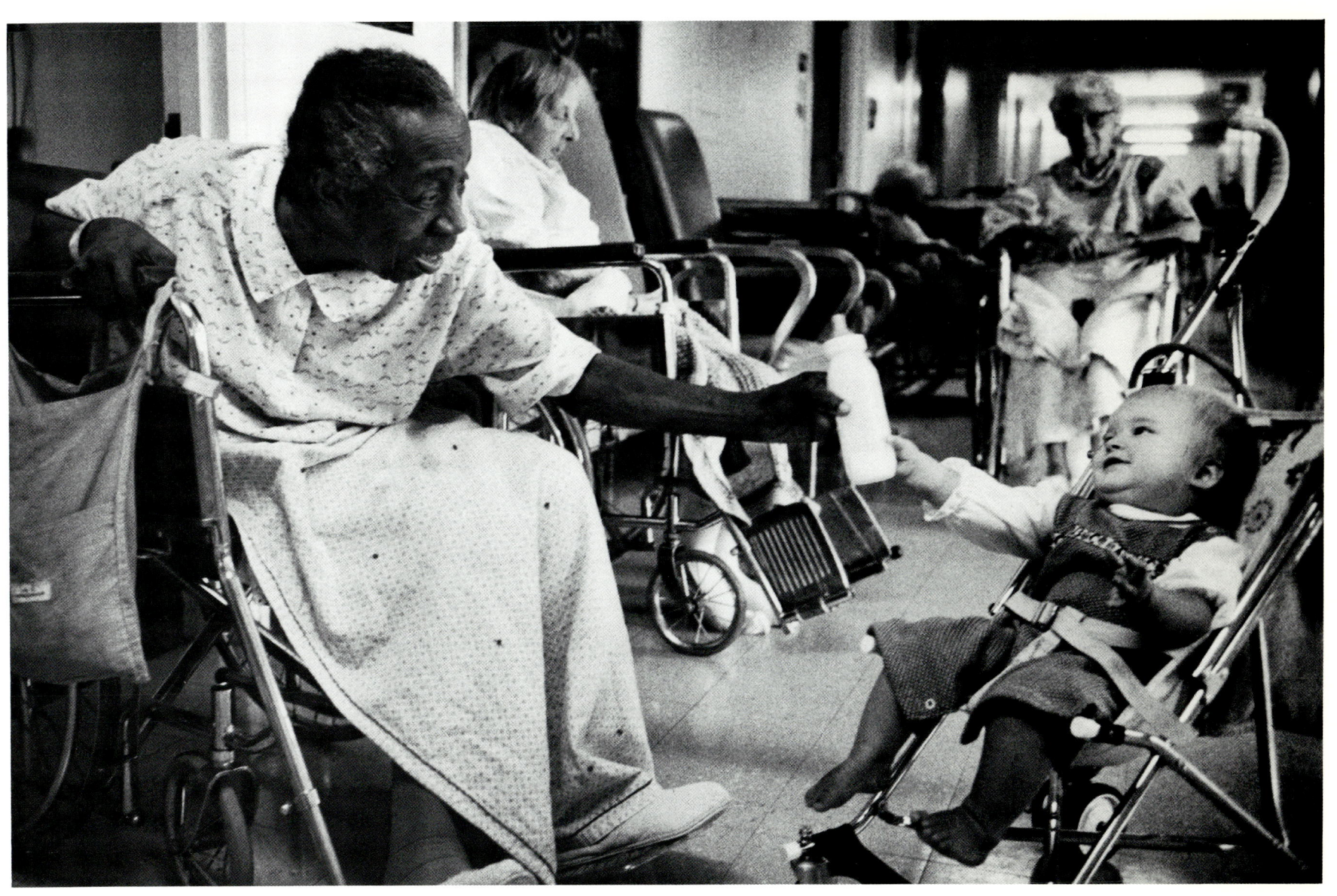

DEATH HATH NO TERROR

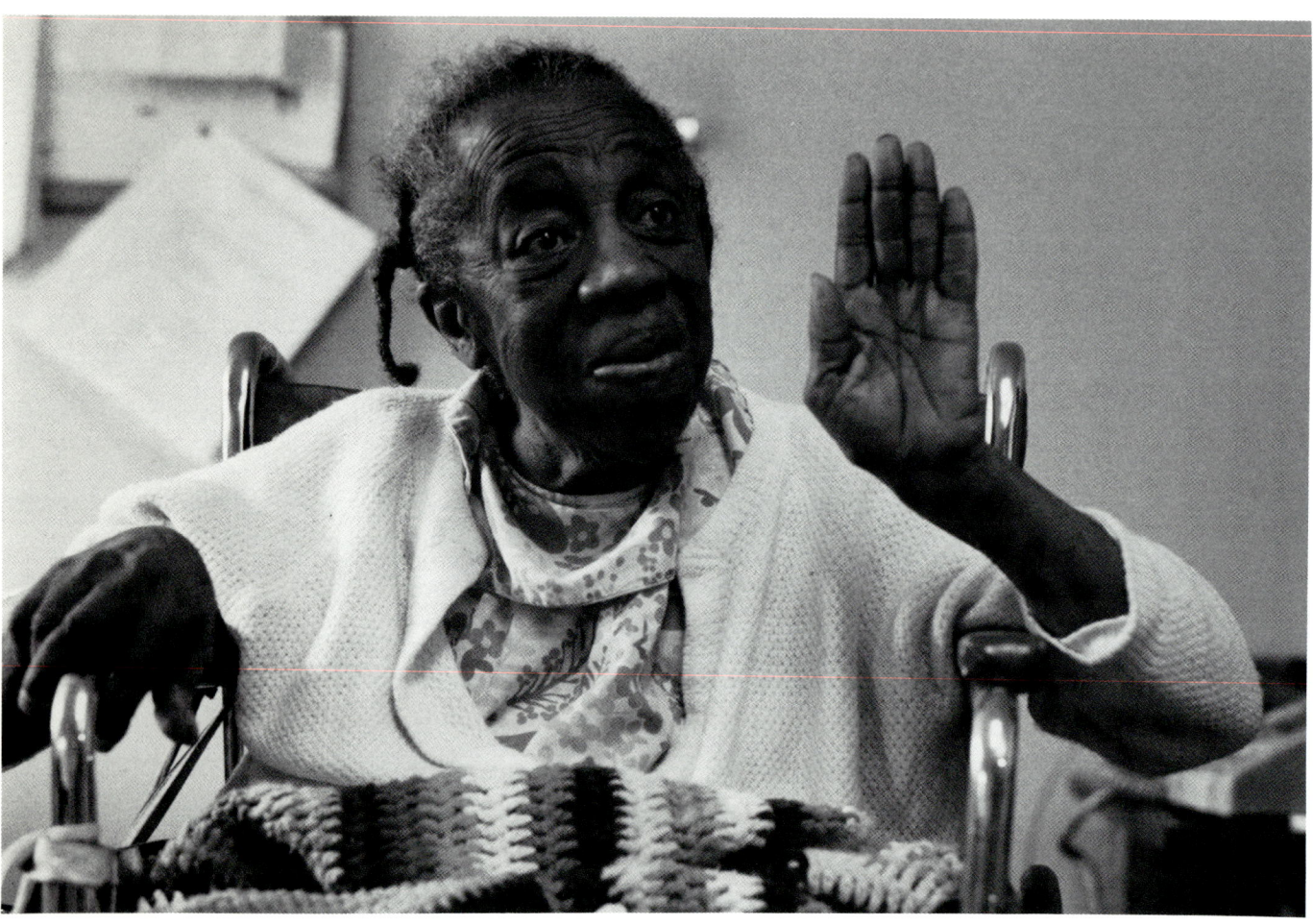

Essie, a spinster, grew up in Salem, Oregon. A fundamentalist Christian for over fifty years, she is a regular at all the religious services at the home and is a stickler for decorum. She will deliver a stern warning to anyone who gets out of hand and has even bottlenecked the aisle to deny access to repeat offenders. I asked her if she ever danced in her life. She gave me a stern look, then her face softened into a slyly amused smile. "Lord no, the only time I ever danced was at the end of my father's switch."

I was the chiefest of sinners, but the Lord chose to save me. He bled and died for me. I had a good Christian mother, but I didn't know anything about salvation until 1925, March 11, 1925, when the Lord filled me with the Holy Ghost and Power. He's been with me ever since and has never let me down. And so I've had a wonderful life.

I guess the Lord put me here at the nursing home for a reason. When I first arrived I was acquainted with a young lady and she was sick, but she was filled with the power of the Holy Ghost. The Lord must have put me here to be with her while she was dying because I didn't have any other reason for being here. When she died I had her blessed with the Holy Spirit.

There are many people here who need to have their understanding opened. I don't preach myself, but I ask the Lord to undertake to open up their understanding. What could I tell someone, except the truth of the Gospel? It's all in the scripture. The Book of Acts II and IV is where to study the Word and receive the Baptist blessing of the Holy Ghost. I'm looking forward to death, because the scripture says, "Death hath no terror . . ." I will leave off to be with the Lord. Amen.

—Essie

MOM REALLY BELIEVED

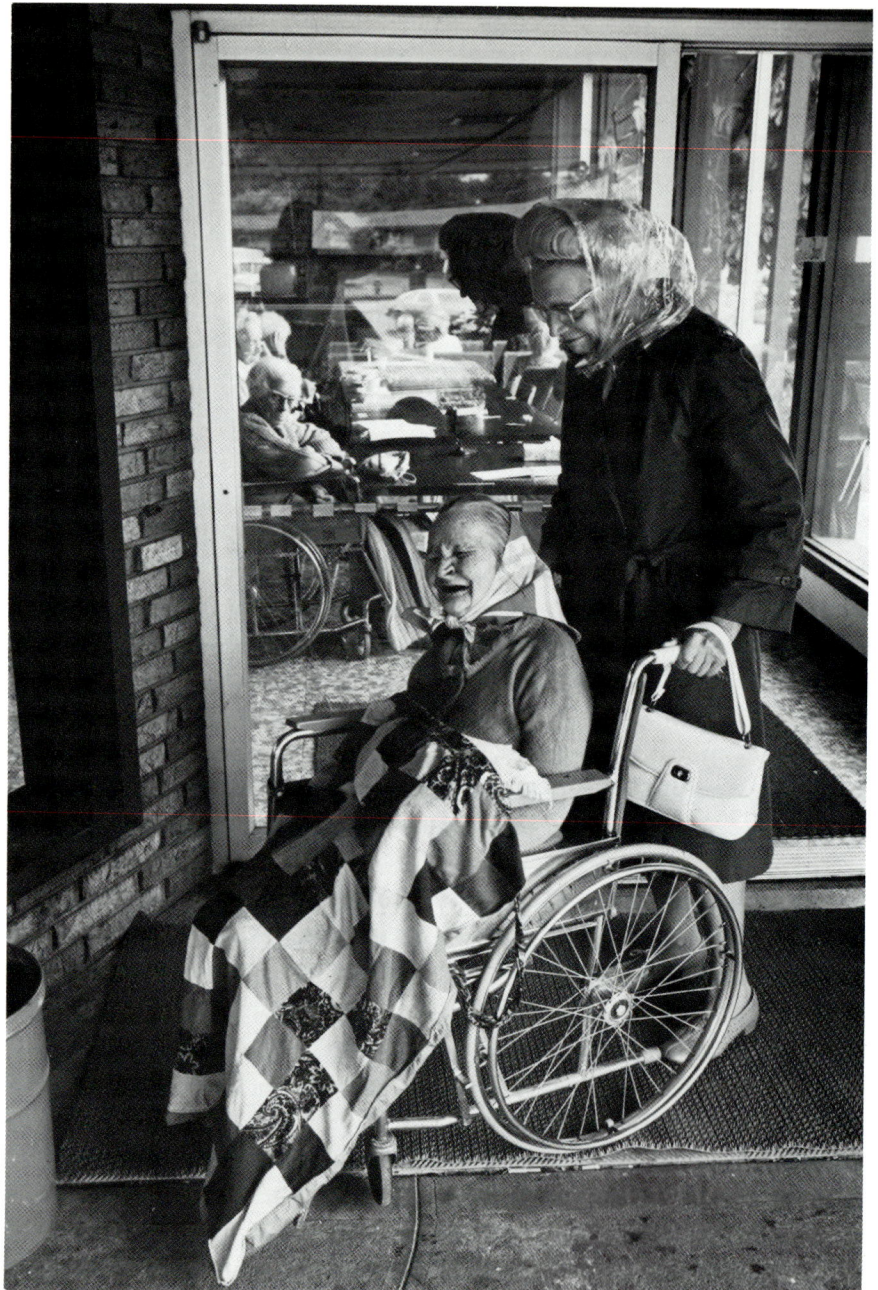

Born into poverty in Barnum, Texas, in 1892, Viola was the eldest of twelve children. The family moved from Texas to Oklahoma and finally settled in Washington state where they cooked for lumber and hop-picker camps. At 18 she married, but her husband's poor health prevented him from supporting the family. Viola scratched out a living by working in commercial laundries and by doing housework.

At 40, she experienced a nervous breakdown, affecting her in such a way that she talked continuously for twelve straight days. She finally pulled out of it, at the same time undergoing a strong religious conversion. She asked the Lord to come into her heart, and her new-found faith provided her an inner peace that sustained her the rest of her life.

Viola's left side was paralyzed by a stroke in 1963, and for the next seventeen years she was confined to different nursing homes. She was always able to feed herself but was otherwise dependent on the staff. I first got to know Viola when I worked as an aide and later as a friend. She always called me Brother Crandall. One early morning I received a phone call from her family at the hospital, saying that Viola was dying and she wanted to say goodbye to me. "Brother Crandall, I'm ready. Jesus, I'm coming home; Jesus, I'm coming home." Six hours later, she died.

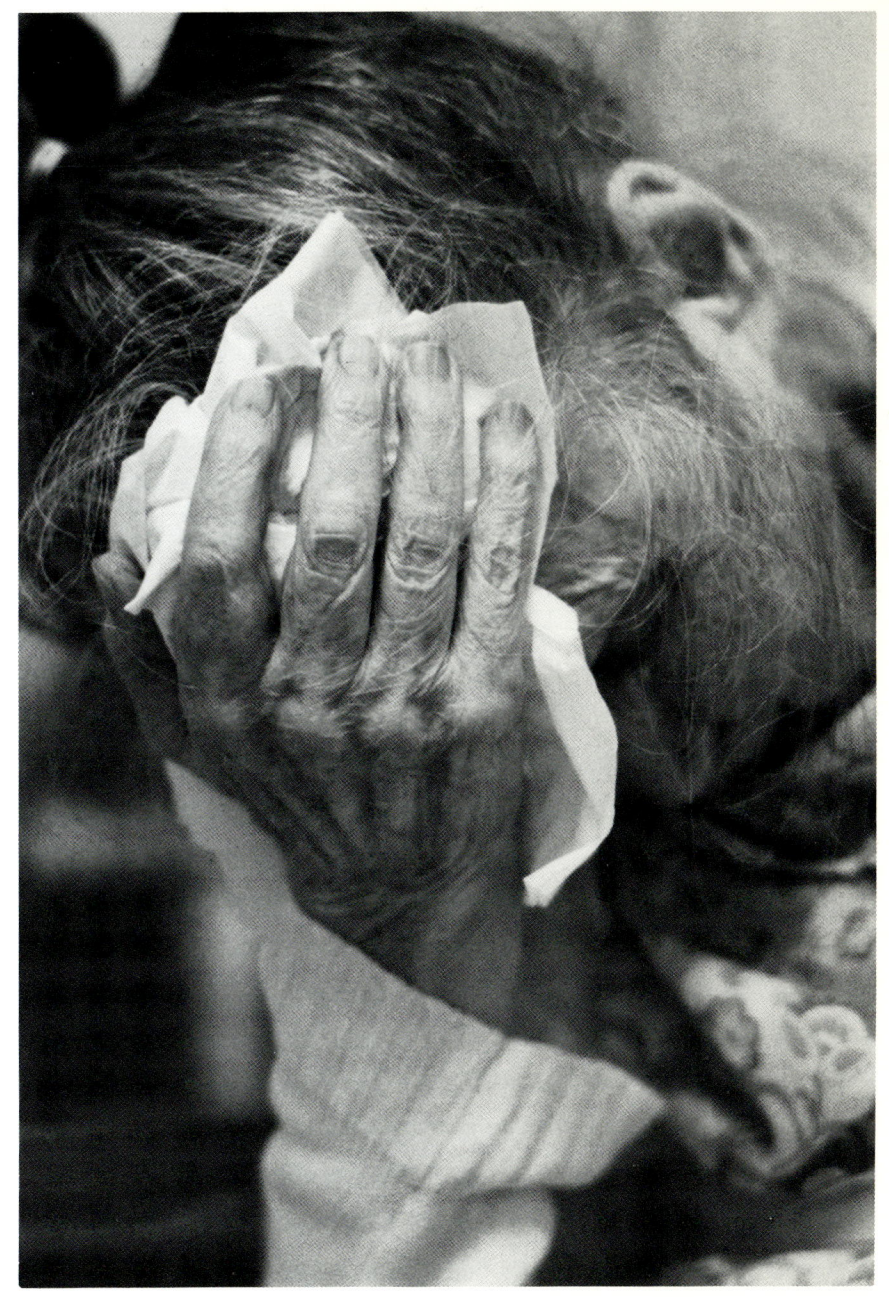

Mom wasn't in any excruciating pain, but she was very uncomfortable. Her hand never stopped hurting—she said that it hurt all the time. She called her discomfort her affliction. "Many are the afflictions of the righteous, but the Lord delivers them out of them all." Mom really believed that. She couldn't hardly see at all, and reading her Bible was impossible. But what she had already read, Mom had stored away. Lots of times when she was sitting there apparently doing nothing, she was praying and going over the scriptures in her mind. I know she did this 'cause one day I was complaining about something and she told me, "Dorothy, there's nothing in the world I can do to help you except pray for you." Isn't that something? To have your Mom say that to you?

About six weeks before she died, I was visiting Mom and she said, "You know, I have lost three roommates. My time is going to come pretty soon." I said, "Oh, come on Mom, let's don't talk like that." Well, she told me, "Now Dorothy, if this situation were reversed and you said that, I would say, "The Lord gave, and the Lord taketh away. Blessed be the name of the Lord." Then she gave a little testimony about how good the Lord had been to her, reciting the Twentieth Psalm where it says, "Surely goodness and mercy shall follow me all the days of my life, and I shall dwell in the house of the Lord forever." Spiritually, she had just steeled herself for whatever was ahead.

—Viola's daughter, Dorothy

RECOVERY

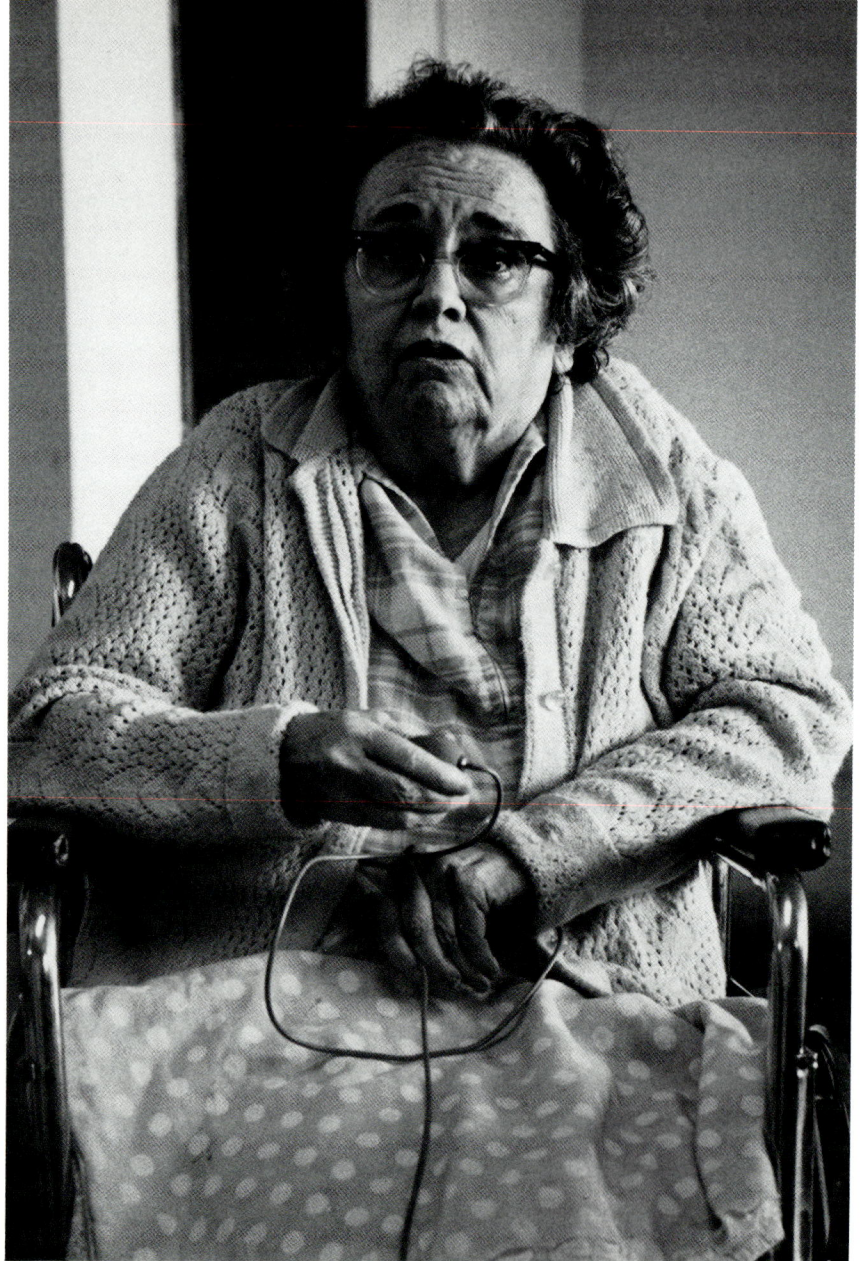

During World War II, Hazel enlisted in the WACS and was assigned to counterintelligence work. With an eye for observation and the unprepossessing air of a matronly school teacher, she excelled in her first major assignment, fronting as a public relations officer in a unit suspected of harboring a spy operation. After the war, she enrolled at the University of California, Berkeley, where she received an M.A. in English literature. She taught high school and college English for three years, then went to work for the Girl Scouts of America, eventually becoming a regional director.

At the nursing home, Hazel maintains an interest in the welfare of other residents. One of her roommates, Jessie—a rugged woman in her nineties who used to raise chickens and who, according to Hazel, "wakes up in the morning swearing like a Marine"—complained about having nothing to do. Hazel prepared a reading list for Jessie, and before long she became an avid reader.

This photograph is Hazel's self-portrait. She titled it, "Recovery."

Your thoughts can do so much, affect the condition of your body. I've known that for a long time, from when I was taking examinations at school. All you need to do is stay relaxed and clear your thinking. I got straight A's all the time and that's how I did it. Wasn't smarter than others, just knew a better technique.

The more difficult the conditions, the greater the challenge, the more it just adds fuel to the fire. I've noticed how progressive my Parkinson's disease is, but it doesn't frighten me at all. I like to know what I'm dealing with. It gets harder to walk, I feel stiffer, and sometimes when I talk it's as though I have marbles in my mouth. I won't let it get the best of me.

I have high ups and low downs and right now I'm at the high cycle. I feel like I could lick a wildcat. But I know it won't last. When you go down into the valley it's correspondingly low. According to the degree I go up, I go down. I get so I don't want to live . . . I think that's about as low as you can get.

When it's hard for me to go on I think about the fact that people have put their faith in me. They come to talk to me about their problems right here in this institution. And it makes me realize how foolish I would be not to snap right out of that state. It's a kind of therapy I can do by myself. It's a change that I don't think a therapist could get out of me.

I'm real pleased with the way things are going on the whole. Things are better than they used to be. I used to be awake all night, every night. I'm better than I was when I came here, and I expect to live and die here, there's no reason I shouldn't, but every day is brighter than the day before. And that's . . . I think that's really something.

—Hazel

I'll Just Whittle Away to Nothing

I don't know much about God or this heaven business, or whether He is or isn't a Supreme Being. I don't know whether He originated from a piss ant or an elephant. Yet I wouldn't commit suicide on account of myself and my children. I'd hate for them to say, "He killed himself." I brought them into this world: two wonderful children, a boy and a girl. I'll just whittle away to nothing than do something that would cause regret for my children.

—Arthur

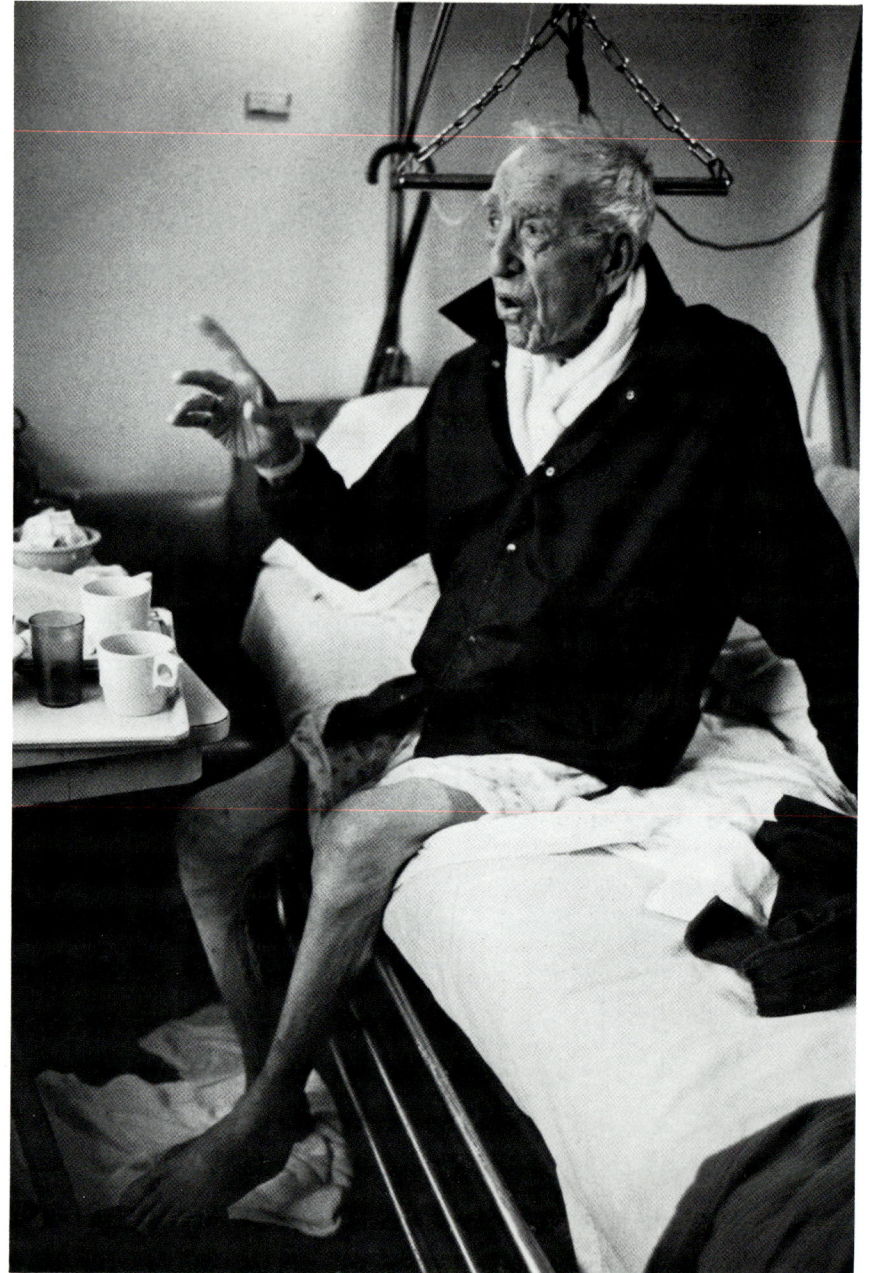

Then Trumpets Sound

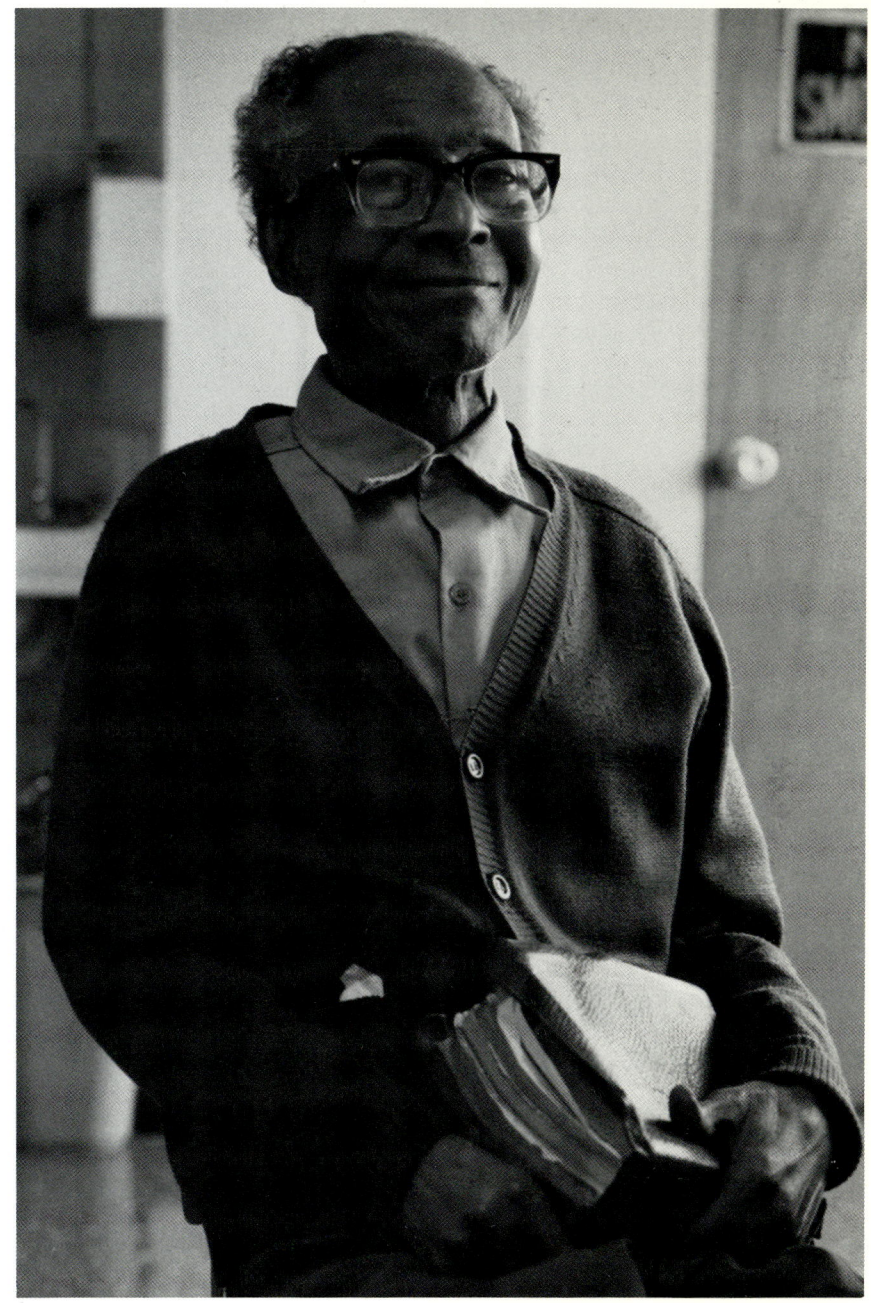

My pastor is the Reverend O. B. Williams. He has been pastoring me for over thirty years at the Vancouver Avenue First Baptist Church. I helped to build that church; I was the secretary of that church; I was licensed and ordained in that church; and I started my ministry in that church.

Before we built the church, we met in a Masonic Lodge in Vancouver, Washington, because we didn't have any other place to worship. We were a little congregation—the Little Church of the Wilderness. Right after World War II we brought ourselves across the Columbia River, just as the children of Israel brought themselves across the Red Sea. We met in the storefront hall where I lived, and we came up with the name Vancouver Avenue Baptist Church. I was elected secretary and held the position until I became ordained and was made Associate Pastor. I carried on with all the duties when Reverend Williams was away: holdin' service, marryin' people, buryin' people.

The church was packed when my wife died, and it will probably be packed when I die. I've requested a short service, but you just don't know. The pastor has control over your funeral. I don't think that I have too much longer to go. I'm seventy-seven and some days I feel like the end is almost here. Lots of people think that when we die we go to heaven right away, but we really only sleep in the grave until Jesus comes back. Then trumpets sound and we are resurrected. That's what I believe.

—Reverend Rogers

THOSE WERE GRANDMA'S QUALITIES

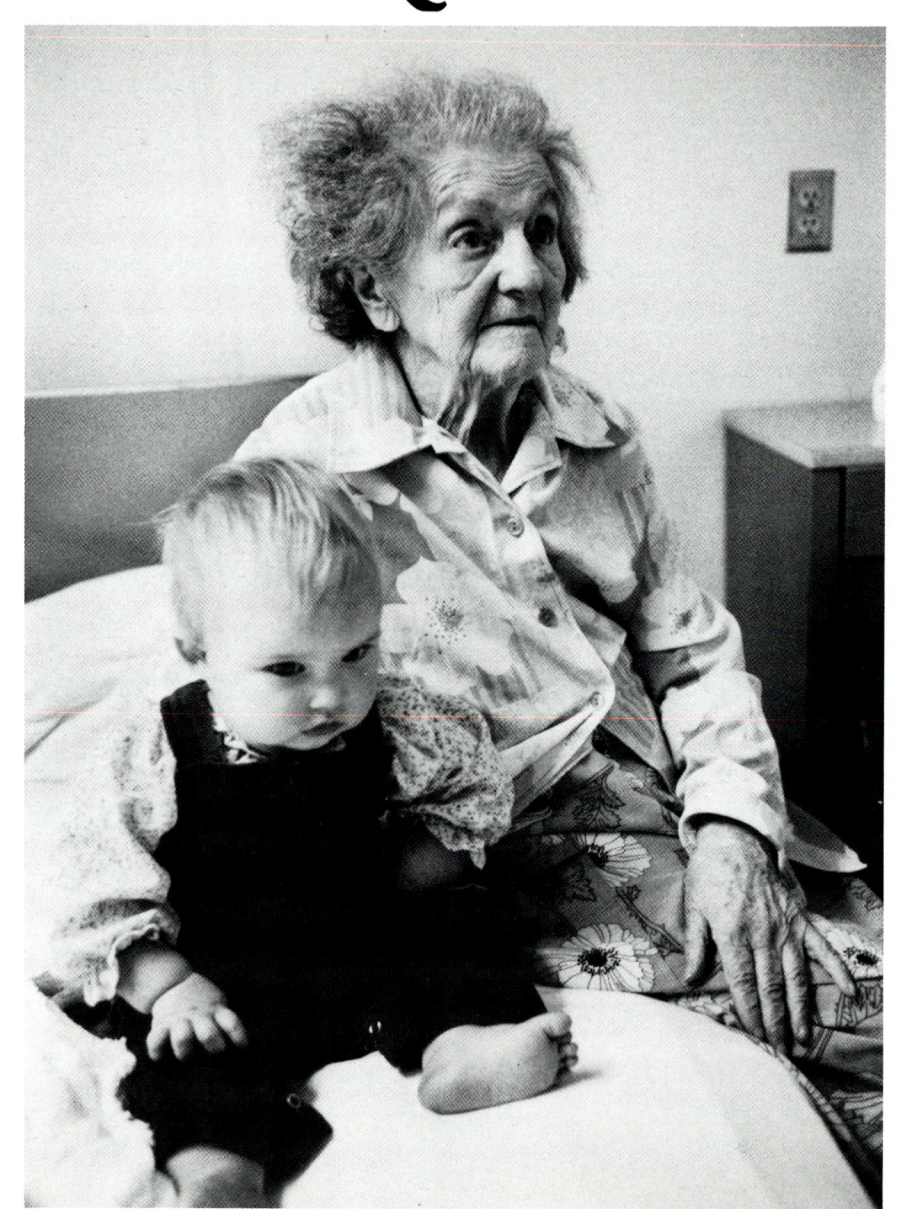

Before Etta died, her granddaughter had made weekly visits and always brought along her baby daughter, Cathryn. She became acquainted with a number of residents and frequently stopped in the hallway to chat with Cathryn's many admirers. Cathryn also appears on the cover of the book, with one of her friends, Essie.

Initially I felt bad about taking my daughter to visit Grandma. As a new parent, you're concerned about cleanliness, and the nursing home isn't a very sanitary place. But I took Cathryn to see her because Grandma loved kids, and she did enjoy seeing Cathryn.

It would have been nice if I had had Cathryn five years earlier, so that she and Grandma could have become friends. It was really impossible for them to establish a family connection. Grandma was senile. And if she had lived for another ten years in the senile state that she was in, how would I have explained to Cathryn that this wasn't the grandmother that Mommy knew? Grandma knew that Cathryn and I were family, but she didn't know how we were related. She had no control over her life. It is difficult to see someone you love that far deteriorated.

I've tried not to romanticize Grandma after her death. But she was the kindest and most generous person that I ever knew. She truly liked everybody. It's very important to me that Cathryn be the kind of person that Grandma was. It gives me great pleasure to see that Cathryn has many of the same nurturing qualities that Grandma had. But I don't want to say, "Cathryn, you become Grandma"—that would be putting a lot of pressure on her. It's more like I'm sitting back and hoping that Grandma's qualities which mean so much to me get passed on to my daughter. Cathryn is such a nurturing child—she takes care of her bears, tucks them into bed, and kisses them goodnight. That gives me great pleasure because those were Grandma's qualities.

—Etta's granddaughter

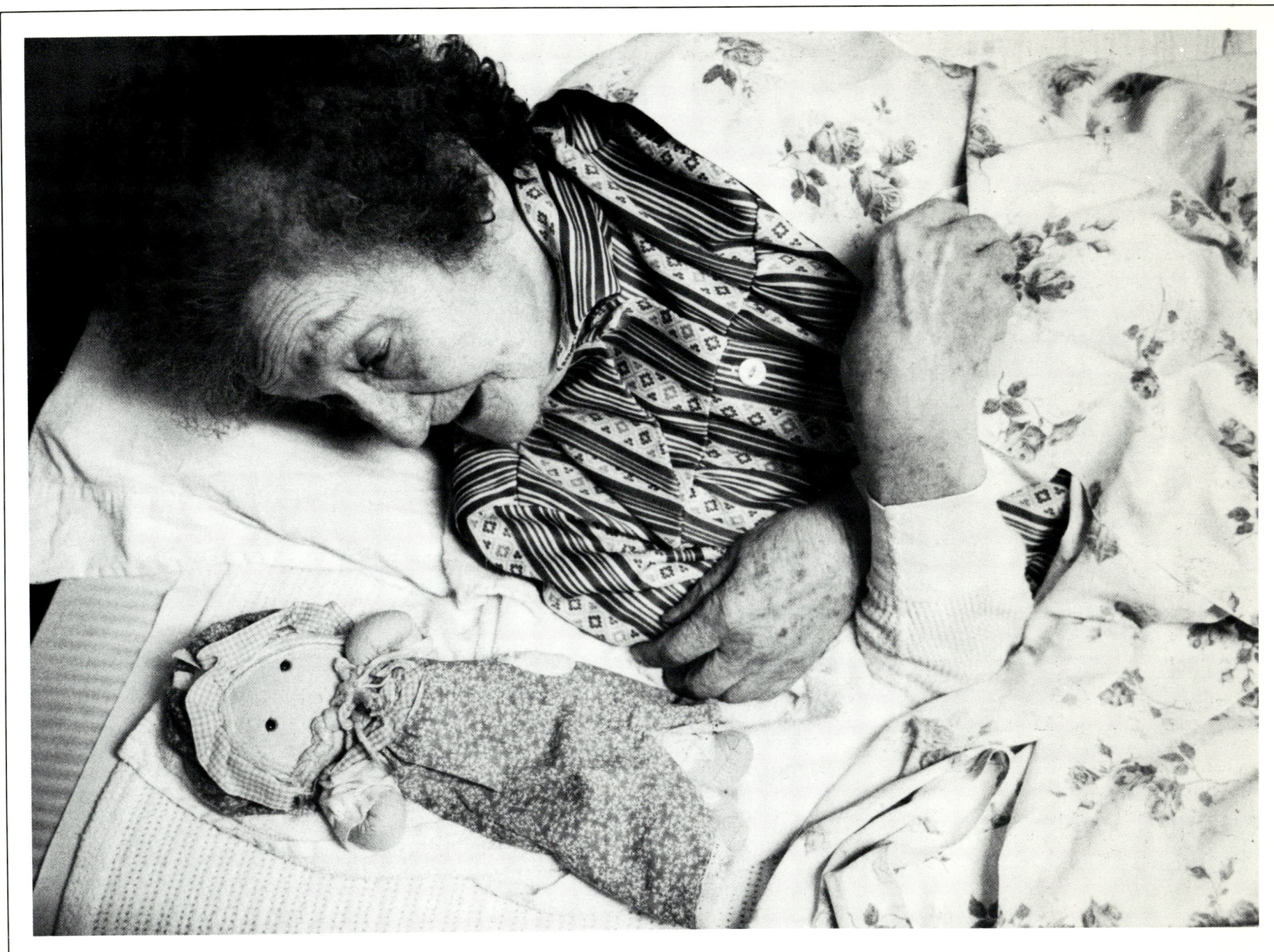

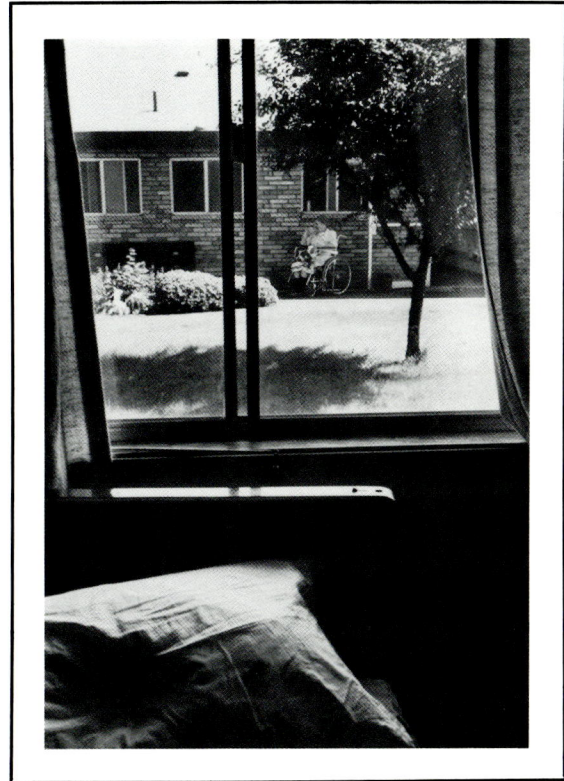

Walter H. Crandall first became interested in the elderly when he was a graduate student at the School of Social Service Administration, University of Chicago, where he worked on a National Science Foundation Project, "Aging and The Aged in the Year 1990: Research Needs." In 1978 he moved to Oregon and became involved with the Gray Panthers' Task Force on Nursing Homes. As part of his work with the Gray Panthers, he wrote *Living In Oregon's Nursing Homes,* a consumer guide. Mr. Crandall lives in Portland, Oregon, with his wife Kathy and daughter Jennifer, and is the leader of his daughter's Girl Scout Troop.

Rob Crandall was born in 1956 in New York and is a graduate of Reed College. He was formerly a free-lance photographer for the Associated Press in Oregon and a staff photographer for the Syracuse Newspapers in New York. He is currently photographing for Picture Group, Inc., an international photography agency. His pictures have appeared in *Life, Newsweek, The New York Times,* as well as many other national and international publications. He lives in Massachusetts with his wife Marie Daly Price.